Palgrave Studies in Public Health Policy Research

Series Editors
Patrick Fafard
University of Ottawa
Ottawa, ON, Canada

Evelyne de Leeuw
University of New South Wales Australia
Liverpool, NSW, Australia

Public health has increasingly cast the net wider. The field has moved on from a hygiene perspective and infectious and occupational disease base (where it was born in the 19th century) to a concern for unhealthy lifestyles post-WWII, and more recently to the uneven distribution of health and its (re)sources. It is of course interesting that these 'paradigms' in many places around the world live right next to each other. Hygiene, lifestyles, and health equity form the complex (indeed, wicked) policy agendas for health and social/sustainable development. All of these, it is now recognized, are part of the 'social determinants of health'.

The broad new public health agenda, with its multitude of competing issues, professions, and perspectives requires a much more sophisticated understanding of government and the policy process. In effect, there is a growing recognition of the extent to which the public health community writ large needs to better understand government and move beyond what has traditionally been a certain naiveté about politics and the process of policy making. Public health scholars and practitioners have embraced this need to understand, and influence, how governments at all levels make policy choices and decisions. Political scientists and international relations scholars and practitioners are engaging in the growing public health agenda as it forms an interesting expanse of glocal policy development and implementation.

Broader, more detailed, and more profound scholarship is required at the interface between health and political science. This series will thus be a powerful tool to build bridges between political science, international relations and public health. It will showcase the potential of rigorous political and international relations science for better understanding public health issues. It will also support the public health professional with a new theoretical and methodological toolbox. The series will include monographs (both conventional and shorter Pivots) and collections that appeal to three audiences: scholars of public health, public health practitioners, and members of the political science community with an interest in public health policy and politics.

More information about this series at
http://www.palgrave.com/gp/series/15414

Benjamin Ewert • Kathrin Loer
Editors

Behavioural Policies for Health Promotion and Disease Prevention

palgrave
macmillan

Editors
Benjamin Ewert
FernUniversität in Hagen
Hagen, Germany

Kathrin Loer
FernUniversität in Hagen
Hagen, Germany

Palgrave Studies in Public Health Policy Research
ISBN 978-3-319-98315-8 ISBN 978-3-319-98316-5 (eBook)
https://doi.org/10.1007/978-3-319-98316-5

Library of Congress Control Number: 2018962495

This Palgrave Pivot imprint is published by the registered company Springer Nature Switzerland AG
The registered company address is: Gewerbestrasse 11, 6330 Cham, Switzerland

For Silja, who makes my life so much healthier.
BE
For Oliver, who keeps an eye on us living not too healthy and makes my life delightful.
KL

Foreword

Prologue: Some Questions About Patient Autonomy

Should patients choose? For those who reject paternalism and who prize freedom, "yes" seems like an obvious answer. Hospitals and doctors frequently think so, emphasising the idea of "patient autonomy"—an idea that can be connected with the central argument in John Stuart Mill's great essay, *On Liberty*.

In recent years, there have been vigorous debates about freedom of choice, paternalism, behavioural economics, individual autonomy and the use of defaults (see, e.g. Conly 2012; Thaler and Sunstein 2008). Invoking recent behavioural findings, some people have argued that because human beings err in predictable ways, and cause serious problems for themselves, some kind of paternalism is newly justified, especially if it preserves freedom of choice, as captured in the idea of "libertarian paternalism" (Sunstein and Thaler 2003). These arguments have evident applications to health-related policies of many kinds. Maybe we have overrated the idea of patient autonomy.

Many doctors and hospitals insist that patients should be asked or allowed to choose, whether or not they would choose rightly—not least when their health and well-being are on the line. For all sides, the opposition between paternalism and active choosing seems stark and plain, and indeed it helps to define all of the existing divisions.

My central goal here is to unsettle that opposition and to suggest that it is often illusory. In many contexts, an insistence on active choosing is a form of paternalism, not an alternative to it. This is emphatically true in the context of health. The central reason is that *some people choose not to choose*. Sometimes they make that choice explicitly (and indeed are willing to pay a considerable amount to people who will choose for them). They have actively chosen not to choose.

Sometimes people (including some patients) have made no explicit choice; they have not actively chosen anything. But it is nonetheless reasonable to infer that in particular contexts, their preference is not to choose, and they would say so if they were asked. They might fear that they will err. They might be aware of their own lack of information or perhaps their own behavioural biases (such as unrealistic optimism). They might find the underlying questions confusing, difficult, painful and troublesome—empirically, morally or otherwise. They might not enjoy choosing. They might be busy and lack "bandwidth" (Mullainathan and Shafir 2013, 39–66). They might not want to take responsibility for potentially bad outcomes for themselves (and at least indirectly for others). They might anticipate their own regret and seek to avoid it. In the medical context, patients might be under considerable stress, and prefer some kind of default rule, or strong suggestion, for exactly that reason.

But even when people prefer not to choose, many doctors, nurses and others favour and promote active choosing on the part of patients, on the ground that it is good for patients to choose. To this extent, active choosing counts as paternalistic. *Choice-requiring paternalism* might be an attractive form of paternalism, but it is no oxymoron, and it is paternalistic nonetheless. That form of paternalism is particularly common in the medical context. In a sense, it overrides patient autonomy, though it purports to operate in the name of that ideal.

If people are *required* to choose even when they would prefer not to do so, active choosing counts as a species of non-libertarian paternalism in the sense that people's own choice not to choose is being rejected. We shall see that in many cases, those who favour active choosing (including doctors) are actually mandating it, and may therefore be overriding (on paternalistic grounds) people's choice not to choose. When people prefer not to choose, required choosing is a form of coercion—though it may be the right form, at least where active choosing does not increase the likelihood and magnitude of errors, and where it is important to enable people to learn and to develop their own preferences.

If, by contrast, people are *asked whether they want to choose*, and can opt out of active choosing (in favour of, say, a default rule), active choosing counts as a form of libertarian paternalism. In some cases, it is an especially attractive form. A doctor might ask people whether they want to make a choice among treatments, or instead rely on the standard approach.

With such an approach, people are being asked to make an active choice between the default and their own preference, and in that sense, their liberty is fully preserved. Call this *simplified active choosing*. Simplified active choosing has the advantage of avoiding the kinds of pressure that come from a default rule, while also allowing people to rely on such a rule if they like. In the future, we should see, and we should hope to see, adoption of this approach by a large number of institutions, both public and private, and it has strong claims for adoption in the medical domain.

Asking Patients

We could easily imagine cases in which people are explicitly asked to choose whether they want to choose. Patients might be asked: *Do you want to make a series of choices, or do you want to be defaulted into those that seem to work best for most people, or for people like you?* In such cases, many people may well decide in favour of a default rule, and thus decline to choose, because of a second-order desire not to do so. They might not trust their own judgement; they might not want to learn. The topic might make them anxious. They might have better things to do. They might want to appoint some kind of surrogate, or to allow for such an appointment.

Simplified active choosing—active choosing, with the option of using a default—has considerable promise and appeal, not least because it avoids at least many of the influences contained in a default rule, and might therefore seem highly respectful of autonomy while also giving people the ability to select the default. Note, however, that simplified active choosing is not quite a perfect solution, at least for those people who genuinely do not want to choose. After all, they are being asked to do exactly that. At least some of those people (including some patients) likely do not want to have to choose between active choosing and a default rule, and hence they would prefer a default rule to an active choice between active choosing and a default rule. Even that active choice takes time and effort, and imposes costs, and some or many people might not want to bother. In this respect, supposedly libertarian paternalism, in the form of an active choice between active choosing and a default, itself has a strong non-libertarian dimension—a conclusion that brings us directly to the next section.

Choice-Requiring Paternalism

Is it paternalistic to require active choosing, when people (e.g. employees or patients) would prefer not to choose? Is it paternalistic for doctors to require people to choose?

To answer these questions, we have to start by defining paternalism. There is of course an immensely large literature on that question (see, e.g. Coons and Weber 2013; Dworkin 1988). Let us bracket the hardest questions and note that while diverse definitions have been given, it seems clear that the unifying theme of paternalistic approaches is that *a private or public institution does not believe that people's choices will promote their welfare, and it is taking steps to influence or alter people's choices for their own good.*

What is wrong with paternalism, thus defined? Those who reject paternalism typically invoke welfare, autonomy or both. They tend to believe that individuals are the best judges of what is in their interests, and of what would promote their welfare, and that outsiders should decline to intervene because they lack crucial information. John Stuart Mill himself emphasised that this is the essential problem with outsiders, including government officials. Mill insisted that the individual "is the person most interested in his own well-being," (Mill 1859) and the "ordinary man or woman has means of knowledge immeasurably surpassing those that can be possessed by any one else" (id.). When society seeks to overrule the individual's judgement, it does so on the basis of "general presumptions," and these "may be altogether wrong, and even if right, are as likely as not to be misapplied to individual cases" (id.). Mill's goal was to ensure that people's lives go well, and he contended that the best solution is for outsiders to allow people to find their own path.

This is an argument about welfare, grounded in a claim about the superior information held by individuals. It very much applies to patients, who have unique access to their own tastes, values, fears, hopes and situations. But there is an independent argument from autonomy, which emphasises that even if people do not know what is best for them, and even if they would choose poorly, they are entitled to do as they see fit (at least so long as harm to others, or some kind of collective action problem, is not involved). On this view, freedom of choice has intrinsic and not merely instrumental value. It is an insult to individual dignity, and a form of infantilisation, to eliminate people's ability to go their own way. The interest in patient autonomy stems in part from an insistence on this point.

Whether or not these objections to paternalism are convincing, there are legitimate questions about whether and how they apply to people whose choice is not to choose. On reflection, they apply quite well, and so choice-requiring paternalism is no oxymoron. People might decline to choose for multiple reasons. They might believe that they lack information or expertise. They might fear that they will err. They might not enjoy the act of choosing; they might like it better if someone else decides for them. They might not want to incur the emotional costs of choosing, especially for situations that are painful or difficult to contemplate (such as organ donation or end-of-life care).

They might find it a relief, and in some contexts even fun, to delegate. They might not want to take responsibility. They might be too busy. They might not want to pay the psychic costs associated with regretting their choice. Active choosing saddles the chooser with responsibility for the choice, and reduces the chooser's welfare for that reason. This point emphatically holds in the medical context.

In daily life, people defer to others, including friends and family members, on countless matters, and they are often better off as a result. In ordinary relationships, people benefit from the functional equivalent of default rules, some explicitly articulated, others not. Within a marriage, for example, certain decisions (such as managing finances or planning vacations) might be made by the husband or wife by default, subject to opt out in particular circumstances. That practice has close analogues in many contexts in which people are dealing with private or public institutions (including hospitals and doctors) and choose not to choose. Indeed, people are often willing to pay others a great deal to make their choices for them. But even when there is no explicit payment or grant of the power of agency, people might well prefer a situation in which they are relieved of the obligation to choose, because such relief will reduce decision costs, error costs or both.

Suppose, for example, that Jones believes that she is not likely to make a good choice about his health care, and that she would therefore prefer a default rule, chosen by someone who is a specialist in the subject at hand. In Mill's terms: Does not Jones know best? Or suppose that Smith is exceedingly busy, and wants to focus on her most important concerns, not on a question about the right approach for her, or even about the right privacy setting on her computer. Does not Mill's argument support respect for Smith's choice? In such cases, the welfarist arguments seem to argue in favour of deference to the chooser's choice, even if that choice is not to choose. If we believe in freedom of choice on the ground that people are uniquely situated to know what is best for them, then that very argument should support respect for people when they freely choose not to choose.

Or suppose that Winston, exercising his autonomy, decides to delegate decision-making authority to someone else, and thus to relinquish the power to choose, in a context that involves his health. Is it an insult to Winston's dignity, or instead a way of honouring it, if a private or public institution refuses to respect that choice?

It is at least plausible to suppose that respect for autonomy requires respect for people's decisions about whether and when to choose. That view seems especially reasonable in view of the fact that people are in a position to make countless decisions, and they might well decide that they would like to exercise their autonomy by focusing on their foremost concerns, not on what seems trivial, boring or difficult.

Paths Forward

Many people have insisted on an opposition between active choosing and paternalism, and in some cases, they are correct to do so. In the domain of health care, active choosing has an important and permanent place. But in many contexts, the opposition is illusory, even a logical error, because people do not want to choose actively. To be sure, the power to choose may well have intrinsic value, but people often exercise that power by delegating authority to others. Nanny states forbid people from choosing, but they also forbid people from choosing not to choose. If and to the extent that hospitals and doctor forbid that choice, they are acting as nannies.

If choice architects are prohibiting people from choosing, they might well be acting paternalistically—and the context of health care, paternalism runs into serious objections on the basis of both autonomy and welfare. But if choice architects *require* people to choose, they may also be acting paternalistically—at least if they are motivated by the belief that active choosing is good and important, notwithstanding the fact that people reject that belief. Insistence on active choosing may simultaneously reduce people's welfare and insult their autonomy—not least when people are vulnerable or aware of their own ignorance, and want some direction and help.

To be sure, active choosing has a central place in a free society, and I have emphasised that it needs to play a large role in the health care system.

But for those involved in that system, as for everyone else, the same concerns that motivate objections to paternalism in general can be applied to paternalistic interferences with people's choice not to choose.

Robert Walmsley University Professor
Harvard University,
Cambridge, MA, USA

Cass R. Sunstein

References

Conly, S. (2012). *Against autonomy. Justifying coercive paternalism.* Cambridge: Cambridge University Press.

Coons, C., & Weber, M. (2013). *Paternalism: Theory and practice.* Cambridge: Cambridge University Press.

Dworkin, G. (1988). *The theory and practice of autonomy.* Cambridge: Cambridge University Press.

Mill, J. S. (1859). *On liberty* (K. Casey, Ed.). 2002.

Mullainathan, S., & Shafir, E. (2013). *Scarcity: Why having too little means so much.* London: Macmillan.

Sunstein, C. R., & Thaler, R. H. (2003). Libertarian paternalism is not an oxymoron. *The University of Chicago Law Review, 70*, 1159–1202.

Thaler, R. H., & Sunstein, C. R. (2008). *Nudge: Improving decisions about health, wealth, and happiness.* New Haven: Yale University Press.

Preface

In an ideal world, public health policymaking would perfectly contribute to keeping citizens healthy—in this ideal world, hardly anybody would become a patient or would need medical treatment. But there is, of course, no such ideal world free from illness and the need for cure. Both public health and health care are needed and together useful to help people to get along with infections, diseases and (too often) hazardous environments, but also to help them to stay as healthy as possible. Both spheres of health policy (public health and health care) are not only generally relevant as such in developed democratic societies, but they also command much attention from political actors and a large budget.

Cass Sunstein's somewhat philosophical perspective on patient's choice and active choosing in general sets as an overture the tone for our book: We focus on policymaking in public health that focuses on individual decision-making, be it of patients or citizens in general. Policymaking in public health more and more tries to influence people's lifestyles, their eating and drinking behaviour, physical activities and so on. Nearly all industrialised countries are far away from the ideal world of a healthy people that is rarely in need of health care. Industrialised countries, their liberal democratic societies and market economies face the dilemma of letting people enjoy the freedom of choice, offering them the broadest range of products and services possible, while simultaneously experiencing the exponential growth of diseases caused by unhealthy lifestyles.

Although we know about the limits of policymaking, we consider politics and policymaking to be highly important for dealing with that dilemma and finding possible solutions that could alleviate the effects of consumerism and libertarian ways of living. Maybe that is why public health becomes ever more relevant on national but also on the international level. This book shall contribute to the debate on current challenges in public health from a political and social science point of view. As political scientists, we look at political, societal and organisational contexts, highlight the significance of actors and incorporate the effect that institutions have on actors and policies. Our view shall be applied on the question how choice architects design people's environments, and if and in which contexts active choosing is adequate when dealing with the challenges of public health policymaking.

Hagen, Germany — Benjamin Ewert
Hagen, Germany — Kathrin Loer

Acknowledgments

We would like to kindly thank Evelyne de Leeuw and Patrick Fafard for their most valuable comments on a previous version of the book's manuscript.

Contents

Notes on Contributors

Benjamin Ewert is a political and social scientist (Postdoctoral Fellow) at the FernUniversität in Hagen. Benjamin's recent research interest is the interplay of (behavioural) public policy and health promotion in settings such as neighbourhoods and schools. He studies also the role of social innovations in (local) welfare systems.

Kathrin Loer is a political scientist (Postdoctoral Fellow) at the FernUniversität in Hagen. She holds a PhD in Social Science from the University of Osnabrück. Working as a political consultant in public health she returned to academia in 2013. Her research focuses on health and consumer policies but also on theoretical topics in public policy. Current research projects aim at linking theoretical and conceptual questions of public policy with empirical research on health and energy policy.

Jessica Pykett is a social and political geographer at the University of Birmingham, where she researches the impacts of behavioural sciences and neurosciences on public policy and chairs the Embodied Geographies research group. She teaches on the spatial politics of welfare, work and wealth.

Holger Strassheim is Professor of Political Sociology at the University of Bielefeld. His work explores the intertwinement of science and politics in world society, the role of expertise in public policy, and the governance networks in and between policy areas. He is co-editor of the Advances in Critical Policy Studies series published by Edward Elgar.

CHAPTER 1

Understanding the Challenges in Public Health Policymaking: Introduction

Kathrin Loer and Benjamin Ewert

Abstract Loer and Ewert introduce the key issues of the book and initiate the discussion on contemporary public health policymaking: they point out how individual and societal parameters interfere with policy interventions. The introduction to the book explains how this idea of reciprocity will be combined with the current debate on struggles against lifestyles being (potentially) dangerous to health. The reader will learn how public health can be conceptualised in the light of the most relevant challenges to policymaking. Furthermore, the introduction gives a brief overview of the following chapters.

Keywords Public health • Contemporary challenges • Policymaking • Individual and societal dimensions

K. Loer (✉)
FernUniversität in Hagen, Hagen, Germany
e-mail: kathrin.loer@fernuni-hagen.de

B. Ewert
FernUniversität in Hagen, Hagen, Germany
e-mail: benjamin.ewert@fernuni-hagen.de

B. Ewert, K. Loer (eds.), *Behavioural Policies for Health Promotion and Disease Prevention*, Palgrave Studies in Public Health Policy Research, https://doi.org/10.1007/978-3-319-98316-5_1

Introduction

'Prevention is better than cure' is a frequently heard truism, and indeed it may seem obvious that preventing a potential or impending problem is far preferable to having to deal with a problem after it has occurred. However, when it comes to public policy, it seems that preventing societal problems is no simple matter, since preventative measures can often conflict with political and social realities and must also contend with a complex tangle of influencing factors. This seems especially true for most issues in public health, which are influenced by both societal and individual factors: for example, even when a person's living environment provides sanitation facilities, infrastructure, information, advice and support for a healthy life, this still does not guarantee that this person will adopt a healthy lifestyle, and the converse is equally true. It is easy to imagine the complexity that is intrinsic to both spheres of public health, whether in relation to communicable diseases or non-communicable diseases (NCDs) such as asthma and diabetes or causes of NCDs such as obesity.

As we will argue in this book, policymakers may seek to break free of budget constraints (at least in part) by re-inventing approaches that aim to address and influence individual lifestyles. Above all, dietary and exercise habits seem to constitute the largest risk factors when it comes to a range of adverse health outcomes. If we were to ignore for a moment the political context and to overlook the values of the liberal twenty-first-century society, it would be easy to envisage the strict prohibitions and orders that policymakers might introduce to ensure that people desisted from unhealthy behaviours and adopted healthier ones. Alternatively, high taxes might be imposed to discourage people from consuming certain products known to pose a health risk (for a systematic overview of the literature on policy instruments, see Chap. 3). But to return to reality, depending on the political context and political culture in the country concerned, these kinds of intervention would not only be politically risky but would also undo some of the key achievements of the liberal democracies in which we live. Of course, we could easily identify the spectrum of policy instruments (Lowi 1972; Vedung 2003; Howlett 2011) which are considered in political science debate. But, we have to link the literature to public health debates (see Chap. 3).

There is also an ethical dimension when it comes to current health policymaking in the sphere of disease prevention and health promotion: who is ultimately responsible for preserving people's health? How much can and should public policymaking seek to promote 'healthy lifestyles' that help to prevent NCDs? And moreover, who should be responsible for deciding what is healthy and what makes people sick? When we analyse the determinants of the health of populations (e.g. Evans et al. 1994), the complex range of factors that influence people's health becomes obvious. Despite such comprehensive knowledge, an often rather simplistic public debate continues to emphasise certain—apparently undisputed—factors that everybody should be able to address in order to prevent NCDs: better nutrition, more physical activity, giving up smoking and the like. However, the question really is at what proximal or distal level of the causation chain policymakers are willing to focus their policy intervention. Is it lifestyle and behaviour, or rather the systems that create the options for lifestyles and behaviours? This book draws from the strand of literature that has already highlighted the imbalanced frequency how policymakers chose between these options in health policy practice. The frequent absence of effective policies for tackling social inequality (Baum and Fisher 2014) is further fuelled by newly emerging and rapidly growing approaches in public health that focus on individual behaviours. The following chapters of this book will acknowledge the reciprocal nature of individual and societal parameters and policy interventions which refer to these parameters. This basic idea will be combined with the current debate on tackling individual lifestyles that constitute a (potential) health risk.

However, before we turn our attention to the question of how policymakers can deal with the complexity involved in public health, we would first like to take a conceptual step back. What do we typically mean by public health? Following Bergenheim et al. (2018) in a first step, we see a difference between public health, national health and population health (Bergenheim et al. 2018, 1), as well as between medicine and health policy. Second, we agree with the important notion that 'health is created largely outside the health sector' (de Leeuw 2017, 330), which means that public health would need methods of engagement across levels, action-logics and governance-policy-action permutations (de Leeuw 2017, 314)—or, to put it differently, 'in the health society health has become a "co-produced" good which needs the cooperation of many sectors and actors in society' (Kickbusch 2007, 158). Additionally, we learn a lot about the differences in conceptualising public health, in particular with regard to political and cultural factors, from this strand of literature (Kananen et al. 2018). Despite interesting national differences in the concept of public health, especially between Nordic countries on the one hand and Western European or North American countries on the other, Kananen et al. (2018) also underline historical changes in the concept of public health. These changes relate to processes of individualisation (active and passive), but they are also strongly linked to the expansion of market mechanisms and the growing relevance of private-sector actors and corporations. This historical research prepares the ground nicely for a better understanding of the challenges of policymaking in public health. The second chapter of this book builds on these findings by exploring and revisiting the assumptions that underlie policymaking in the field of health promotion. Ewert develops a comprehensive and balanced approach to health promotion that integrates the ideas of behavioural sciences. The chapter explains how behavioural insights could be a useful tool in future health promotion policy.

In line with Kananen et al. (2018), and having reviewed a broad swathe of literature, we can attest that the field of public health policy has a number of challenges to contend with, included blurred concepts, a constantly changing environment and the complex tangle of factors that can influence individual health. Factors that affect health and cause diseases do not stop at frontiers. They are independent of administrative levels and do not conform to the idea of policy areas. They therefore demand comprehensive solutions in policymaking. The prevention of diabetes, for example, seems to be resistant to quick-fix solutions since it relates to contemporary living environments (e.g. walkability), food supply and nutrition, education, working routines and many more societal and individual factors, many of which are closely intertwined. The issue of diabetes illustrates the host of issues in public health—particularly with regard to NCDs—that policymakers are now confronted with. However, political actors at various levels are seeking policies that can help prevent disease and promote health.

In a comprehensive perspective, Nancy Milio (1981) outlined how health can be promoted through public policy and presented her analysis of the USA. Her study laid the groundwork for future work on public health promotion and yielded insights that continue to play a decisive role in current debates: Milio unveils a spectrum of obstacles that help explain why a comprehensive approach to disease prevention and health promotion was still missing. She pointed out that a 'clear health policy goal' was absent and that political actors lack responsibility and accountability with regard to 'health-making policy options' (Milio 1981, 207). We find a large number of promising individual studies in public health, as well as a small but very significant research literature that takes a public policy perspective on public health (e.g. Clavier and de Leeuw 2013; Fafard 2015), which are very instructive as successors to Milio's comprehensive study.

The literature on public health and the welfare state generally describes a variety of challenges that nearly all developed welfare states have to contend with. Generally speaking, shrinking budgets for social policy, at least in some high-income countries such as Canada, Germany or the UK (OECD 2014), are forcing institutional changes, and it seems as if many stakeholders in social policy are struggling simply to keep their heads above water. The strong path dependency of social institutions limits the scope for political action and the limits of cross-country policy learning are well known (Korpi 2001; Wood and Gough 2006). This is particularly the case when we look at healthcare systems which focus to a great extent on policies for the delivery of healthcare (e.g. hospitals, doctors, medicines, access issues) instead of *policies for health*. Similarly, we see comparable challenges and problems when we cast our eyes across the different health systems of OECD countries: demographic change, a sharp rise in the incidence of NCDs, as well as technological and medical progress. These three factors are causing acute pressure on health budgets. Besides the severe funding issue, normative and ethical factors are leading to the assumption that public institutions have a moral duty to tackle public health issues. The latter has been re-emphasised by high-level NCD deliberations commissioned by the United Nations that recently lead to the adoption of a resolution (UN 2018) and the WHO Independent High-Level Commission on Noncommunicable Diseases (WHO 2018). However, a normative debate on public health also comes up against dilemmas when it comes to prioritising health goods (Ruger 2004) and illustrates the challenges that policymakers face at all political levels.

Health policies relate to disease prevention and health promotion. These policies result from the fact that, of course, one of the foremost duties of a government is to protect its citizens and safeguard public health. There is a long and controversial academic discussion in public health concerning whether upstream, midstream or downstream interventions are best suited to achieving this aim (for an overview see Frieden 2010), which often results in either individualistic or societal interventions. In contrast to this dichotomy, a working compromise seemed to have been struck in the aftermath of the Ottawa Charter (1986), and this is essential to more recent efforts to promote 'health in all policies' approaches: policymakers (at least in Western countries) have focused on 'intersectoral action', 'healthy public policies' and the 'social determinants of health' in order to shape health-promoting life worlds that support people in adopting 'healthy lifestyles' (McQueen et al. 2012). However, this complementary approach, which has been driven by values such as empowerment, participation and civic engagement, is not carved in stone but simply represents the dominant policy of a specific period of time. Meanwhile, policymakers may revise their strategies for public health in the face of new health challenges—with the struggle against NCDs foremost among these challenges. Political actors need to develop policies that are effective in an increasingly individualistic society, where a wide variety of lifestyles can influence people's state of health. The twentieth-century story of public health suggests that regulation was and is a relatively effective policy instrument for achieving public health goals. In fact, conventional policy instruments such as taxing sugar sweetened beverages do make a difference (e.g. Nakhimovsky et al. 2016). However, the classical spectrum of policy instruments would only be effective if fully applied—often strict regulation (authority) or incentives (see Chap. 3) do make a difference (e.g. taxing sugar sweetened beverages). But many governments are reluctant to use these two instruments but only apply forms of information, capacity building or organisational tools which turns out to be (for the most part) insufficient when it comes to recent public health problems such as NCDs. Of course, one could claim that this has also relates to the absence of strategies that address the social determinants of health (cp. Ewert in this book see Chap. 2). Although instruments play a decisive role in public health, the standard literature (starting with Lowi 1972; Vedung 2003; Howlett 2011; for a comprehensive overview, see Chap. 3) has not so far addressed policy instruments in a systematic way and has not explained the mechanisms by which they operate. The third chapter reveals the ways in which policy instruments work in public health and suggests how to handle, in conceptual terms, policy instruments that are informed by insights from behavioural science. This chapter presents some ideas on how public health can benefit from behavioural insights, on the basis of various empirical examples.

Behavioural policy approaches emanating from the theory of *libertarian paternalism* are currently the focus of much public attention, as it is underpinned by a rapidly expanding scholarly literature (see e.g. John 2018; Hanoch and Barnes 2017). 'Nudges' and 'default choices' (Sunstein and Thaler 2009) are intended to guide people towards healthier lifestyles and are currently being widely promoted. Unsurprisingly, behavioural experts are increasingly advising governments to promote these apparently 'simple' or 'innocent' solutions to tackle various policy problems—especially in relation to the (in fact, highly complex) challenge of preventing NCDs. Prominent examples include 'Nudge Units' set up in the United Kingdom, as well as in many other countries around the world (for a detailed overview, see Botzem and Strassheim 2016). These units sometimes work at arm's length from governments but could also be found as forms of bottom-up approaches (e.g. France, Italy). They have in common that they are exploring strategies for influencing people's behaviour without diminishing their overall freedom in lifestyle choices. Criticised as 'governance by stealth', those policies stand in marked contrast to previous health promotion strategies, which were based on individual empowerment and participation. This book offers insights into various empirical cases from all over the world. The fourth chapter, by Pykett, described how the increasing focus on lifestyle and behavioural approaches in public health policy is affecting other drivers of public health and health inequalities. The chapter develops an alternative approach to analysing behavioural public health policies and their geographic variation, and also considers the active role of place and practices in shaping public health. Furthermore, the chapter presents an idea on how to consider practice-based and sociological accounts of health. The following chapter (Strassheim and Loer) highlights the degree of complexity that has come to characterise the relationship between policymakers and epistemic authority. It focuses particularly on the multiplicity of actors at various levels of public health policymaking, revealing multiple and contradictory dynamics. The example of the International Life Science Institute could be understood as paradigmatic, helping to illustrate how science and private actors can become intertwined to produce 'evidence-based policy'. How evidence-based policy goes on to influence public health will be shown in the fifth chapter.

To summarise, this book focuses on public policymaking on disease prevention and health promotion and takes up earlier movements 'calling for the adoption of healthier life-styles' (Evans et al. 1994, 320). Nevertheless, we consider the spectrum of approaches in the public health debate that range from rather simplistic approaches that level the path from systems-based health promotion to more behaviourist and individual population health (for an overview, see Rootman et al. 2017 on Canada). The second chapter of the book presents a comprehensive view of the various factors that can influence how public policy promotes health

(Chap. 2). Thus, this edited volume benefits from a strong analytical focus on public policymaking in the field of health promotion and suggests a typology of policy instruments that can accommodate behavioural insights (Chap. 3) since such behavioural inputs can empirically be found in public health policymaking. Two current developments are considered as playing the lead role in this regard: (1) the growing need for policies that help to reduce or at least stabilise the rising incidence of NCDs and (2) the rapidly growing trend towards behavioural policymaking, its impact on public policies that try to steer individuals and their lifestyle choices and its interplay with other policy interventions. From this starting point, the book applies a broad perspective to public health promotion, beyond a rather narrow academic perspective; however, at the same time, it seeks not to overestimate the impact of behaviourally informed policymaking. Moreover, it contributes to the current debate that involves governments and authorities at all levels, from the local level to the supra- and international level (Chap. 5).

This contribution aims to develop a theoretical understanding of how policymakers are choosing to address health challenges, how these choices are changing over the course of time and which policy approaches are being applied to meet these challenges. One major goal is to demonstrate how (i.e. based on which underlying assumptions) policymakers put the 'health problems' that have been identified and their assumed causes onto the political agenda. Against the backdrop of these theoretical insights, the empirical chapters (Chaps. 4 and 5) describe and explain how political systems around the world are dealing with these challenges.

References

Baum, F., & Fisher, M. (2014). Why behavioural health promotion endures despite its failure to reduce health inequities. *Sociology of Health & Illness, 36*(2), 213–225.

Bergenheim, S., Edman, J., Kananen, J., & Wessel, M. (2018). Conceptualising public health: An introduction. In J. Kananen, S. Bergenheim, & M. Wessel (Eds.), *Conceptualising public health: Historical and contemporary struggles over key concepts* (pp. 1–17). Oxon/New York: Routledge.

Botzem, S., & Strassheim, H. (2016). *On her majesty's service? The behavioural insights team and its role in the global rise of behavioural change policies.* Paper presented at the 44th ECPR Joint Sessions 2016, Workshop No. 2: Behavioural Change and Public Policy, Pisa, Italy.

Clavier, C., & de Leeuw, E. (2013). *Health promotion and the policy process.* Oxford: Oxford University Press.

de Leeuw, E. (2017). Engagement of sectors other than health in integrated health governance, policy, and action. *Annual Review of Public Health, 38*(1), 329–349.

Evans, R. G., Barer, M. L., & Marmor, T. R. (1994). *Why are some people healthy and others not? The determinants of the health of populations.* Berlin/New York: Walter de gruyter.

Fafard, P. (2015). Beyond the usual suspects: Using political science to enhance public health policy making. *Journal of Epidemiology and Community Health, 69*(11), 1129–1132.

Frieden, T. R. (2010). A framework for public health action: The health impact pyramid. *American Journal of Public Health, 100*(4), 590–595.

Hanoch, Y., & Barnes, A. J. (Eds.). (2017). *Behavioral economics and healthy behaviors: Key concepts and current research.* New York: Routledge.

Howlett, M. (2011). *Designing public policies. Principles and instruments.* Abingdon: Routledge.

John, P. (2018). *How far to nudge? Assessing behavioural public policy.* Cheltenham/ Northampton: Edward Elgar.

Kananen, J., Bergenheim, S., & Wessel, M. (2018). *Conceptualising public health: Historical and contemporary struggles over key concepts.* Oxon/New York: Routledge.

Kickbusch, I. (2007). Health governance: The health society. In D. V. McQueen, I. Kickbusch, & L. Potvin (Eds.), *Health and modernity: The role of theory in health promotion* (pp. 144–161). Berlin: Springer.

Korpi, W. (2001). Contentious institutions: An augmented rational-action analysis of the origins and path dependency of welfare state institutions in western countries. *Rationality and Society, 13*(2), 235–283.

Lowi, T. J. (1972). Four systems of policy, politics, and choice. *Public Administration Review, 32*(4), 298–310.

McQueen, D., Wismar, M., Lin, V., Jones, C. M., & Davies, M. (2012). *Intersectoral governance for health in all policies: Structures, actions and experiences* (Observatory Studies Series 26). Copenhagen: WHO Regional Office for Europe.

Milio, N. (1981). *Promoting health through public policy.* Philadelphia: F. A. Davis Company.

Nakhimovsky, S. S., Feigl, A. B., Avila, C., O'Sullivan, G., Macgregor-Skinner, E., & Spranca, M. (2016). Taxes on sugar-sweetened beverages to reduce overweight and obesity in middle-income countries: A systematic review. *PLoS One, 11*(9), e0163358.

OECD. (2014). *Social expenditure update – Social spending is falling in some countries, but in many others it remains at historically high levels.* Retrieved June 14,

2018, from https://www.oecd.org/els/soc/OECD2014-SocialExpenditure_Update19Nov_Rev.pdf
Rootman, I., Pedersen, A., Frohlich, K., & Dupéré, S. (2017). Health promotion in Canada. In *New perspectives on theory, practice, policy, and research* (4th ed.). Toronto/Vancouver: Canadian Scholars.
Ruger, J. P. (2004). Health and social justice. *Lancet, 364*(9439), 1075.
Thaler, R. H., & Sunstein, C. R. (2009). *Nudge. Improving decisions about health, wealth, and happiness.* New York: Penguin.
United Nations (UN). (2018). Scope, modalities, format and organization of the third high-level meeting of the General Assembly on the prevention and control of non-communicable diseases. *Resolution adopted by the General Assembly on 12 April 2018.* Retrieved June 14, 2018, from http://www.who.int/ncds/governance/third-un-meeting/A-RES-72-274.pdf?ua=1
Vedung, E. (2003). Policy instruments: Typologies and theories. In M.-L. Bemelmans-Videc, R. C. Rist, & E. Vedung (Eds.), *Carrots, sticks & sermons. Policy instruments and their evaluation* (pp. 21–58). New Brunswick: Transaction Publishers.
Wood, G., & Gough, I. (2006). A comparative welfare regime approach to global social policy. *World Development, 34*(10), 1696–1712.
World Health Organization (WHO). (2018). *Time to deliver: Report of the WHO Independent high-level commission on noncommunicable diseases.* Geneva: World Health Organization Licence: CC BY-NC-SA 3.0 IGO.

CHAPTER 2

Underlying Assumptions in Health Promotion Policymaking

Benjamin Ewert

Abstract This chapter explores and revisits the assumptions that underlie policymaking in the field of health promotion. It starts by clarifying what is meant by the term 'underlying assumptions' in the field of health promotion and disease prevention. Subsequently, the central concepts of how public health may be improved will be recapitulated in terms of their underlying assumptions and contrasted with the recent shift towards behavioural principles as applied in health promotion. By examining what a comprehensive approach that reconciles structural and behavioural interventions could look like, the role of behavioural insights in health promotion will be clarified. The chapter ends with some final remarks on future challenges in health promotion policy.

Keywords Health promotion • Social determinants of health • Behavioural interventions • Health nudges • Policymaking

B. Ewert (✉)
FernUniversität in Hagen, Hagen, Germany
e-mail: benjamin.ewert@fernuni-hagen.de

B. Ewert, K. Loer (eds.), *Behavioural Policies for Health Promotion and Disease Prevention*, Palgrave Studies in Public Health Policy Research, https://doi.org/10.1007/978-3-319-98316-5_2

Introduction

According to the World Health Organization (WHO 2017), more than 650 million adults—that is, 13% of the world's adult population—were obese in 2016. Even more worryingly, a new generation of abnormally oversized people are growing up, with over 41 million children aged 0–5 being overweight or obese. As is widely known, obesity is a major risk factor for non-communicable diseases (NCDs) such as cardiovascular diseases, diabetes, and (some) cancers. Despite these rather shocking statistics, the WHO ends its report with the somewhat reassuring remark that 'obesity is preventable' (ibid.). Hence, for health policymakers, how to prevent global epidemics such as obesity is a crucial question. In this chapter, I argue that the answers to this question are far from straightforward and emanate from policymakers 'assumptive worlds' (Klein and Marmor 2012a, 2)—an imaginary set of 'theories about the causes of the problems (…) and about the appropriate solutions' (ibid.) that policymakers draw from when designing policies.

With respect to the challenge posed by obesity, the available health policy options differ significantly in terms of their underlying assumptions: since overeating has an obvious behavioural component—individuals are free to choose healthier foods and eat less—policymakers are inclined to intervene on the individual level. However, instead of addressing 'lifestyle-focused health culprits' (Quigley 2013, 620), policymakers could also pursue societal interventions that focus on the *causes* of unhealthy behaviours. In this case, the problem is not assumed to be the individual who consumes too much fatty or sugary food, but the social environments that entice people to make unhealthy food choices. Irrespective of the level of health policy interventions, the selection of policy instruments has an assumptive component too: should bans, taxes or nudges be used to combat obesity? In all cases, governments' policy choices are inevitably normative, values-based and driven by 'underlying political beliefs and values (…) exerting a significant influence on public health and health promotion policy' (Baum and Fisher 2014, 217). Considered unemotionally, it can be stated that health policy interventions are significantly affected by a policy-research-practice *divide* (Cairney and Oliver 2017).

This chapter explores and revisits the assumptions that underlie policymaking in the field of health promotion. It starts by clarifying what is meant by the term 'underlying assumptions' in the field of health promotion and disease prevention. Subsequently, the central concepts of how public health may be improved will be recapitulated in terms of their underlying assumptions and contrasted with the recent shift towards behavioural principles as applied in health promotion. By examining what a comprehensive approach that reconciles structural and behavioural interventions could look like, the role of behavioural insights in health promotion will be clarified. The chapter ends with some final remarks on future challenges in health promotion policy.

Underlying Assumptions Concerning the Causes of Disease and How Best to Promote Health

Public policymaking can be described as the art of finding new and timely solutions for old problems. According to Peters and Zittoun (2016, 12) '[m]ost of the fundamental questions about public policy that we ask today are those that have been asked for years and even decades'. How to promote and maintain public health is certainly one of those questions, and revolves around related issues such as *Who is to be deemed responsible when it comes to risk avoidance?* and *What is the role of government in health promotion?* As shown in this section, analysing the assumptions that underlie health promotion can provide answers to these recurring dilemmas. However, two preliminary remarks ought to be made: First, there are sound arguments that *health* creates an additional dimension to policymaking. Carpenter (2012, 35) has shown that health politics are indeed different to other policy fields, foremost due to its 'equality and justice claims'. Second, when we speak about underlying assumptions in health promotion, we refer to two distinguishing features which are closely linked to each other: firstly, the degree to which policymakers pursue behavioural or structural interventions, that is, whether the relevant policies take place at the individual level and/or the societal level. Basically, this distinction could be applied for all health promotion policies.

Second, policymakers choose health promotion policies from a range of available options, and pursuing one particular policy strategy always involves rejecting an alternative option. With regard to both features, policymakers' decisions emanate from conscious and often political-ideological preferences for or against specific policies (Raphael 2011, 2014). These preliminary decisions are labelled as *underlying assumptions* in this chapter. Moreover, the policy preferences that dominate can seem largely immune to scientific evidence regarding the real impact of multifaceted health determinants (Baum and Fisher 2014) or, as recent behavioural public policies demonstrate, are fed by selective rather than comprehensive evidence (Strassheim and Korinek 2016). In practice, then, the underlying assumptions of health policymakers are largely shaped by ideological beliefs on how to promote public health (and how not to). This being the case, the next question is: on what normative basis do policymakers select one approach to health promotion over another?

In this regard, Hagen Kühn's (1993) explanatory model of a 'normative aetiology', developed for a study on 'healthism' (Crawford 1980) in the United States, is a useful starting point for further analysis. The term *aetiology*, borrowed from the field of medicine, provides four major reasons why people become ill: (1) pathogens and genetic conditions; (2) individual unhealthy behaviours; (3) factors emerging from the physical environment; and (4) social conditions and relations. The *normative* dimension of the aetiology refers to different levels of social acceptance of the various causes of disease and illness. As a basic rule, the probability that public policy will respond to one of these four causes of disease diminishes progressively as one moves further down the list outlined above—from very high (1) to very low (4). Hence, Kühn's compelling argument is that 'certain factors, causes and conditions seem to have a much better chance of being addressed and researched than others' (Kühn 1993, 130). For example, health risks caused by viral infections such as bird flu are much more likely to be addressed than those caused by inequality of living conditions. Following the model, whether approaches to health promotion 'receive political consideration, gain social acceptance, or appear scientifically respectable' (Lemke 2013, 82) depends much on political interests. Policymakers' *preferred* assumptions, that is, those that shape their mind-set and actions when designing health policies, are heavily influenced by 'power relations in society' (ibid., 83). What is more, Kühn's normative aetiology corresponds well with the dominant biomedical paradigm. The latter explains disease through rather simple causes-and-effects relationships that 'fail to consider the complexity and interrelatedness of social systems' (Spotswood 2016, 6). Accordingly, there is a strong tendency to assume that pathogens and individual behaviours are the most important causes for diseases, while the impact of social problems on health is underplayed (or even neglected). Thus, policymakers do not select and apply a specific health promotion concept on the basis of its 'internal consistency or scientific truth' (Lemke 2013, 83), but with regard to its overall compatibility with society's dominant rationales and social norms. In this *survival of the fittest* contest, health promotion policies that lead to the '[least] resistance or the biggest forbearance' (Kühn 1993, 128) towards social conditions and power relations are the most likely to be selected.

Without explicitly referring to it, contemporary critical health policy analysts confirm the essence of Kühn's normative aetiology. For example, Raphael (2011) identifies—mainly in the Canadian context—seven discourses on the social determinants of health (such as income, education, employment or housing) and ranked these on the basis of their implications for political action. Carter (2015, 380) concludes from a US case study on a local health promotion initiative that 'addressing underlying 'social determinants' of health is a political non-starter'. Consequently, policymakers' strong tendency 'to base their health-promotion policies on behaviourism' (Baum and Fisher 2014, 217) provides fertile ground for new forms of behavioural health promotion such as nudging (see section 'Nudge-Based Health Promotion: Game Changer or More of the Same?').

To sum up, the underlying assumptions concerning the causes of diseases and how to promote health vary widely. As a result, policymaker's selection—or deliberate neglect—of specific health promotion strategies is often ideologically motivated. Above all, 'a strong commitment to neoliberalism' (ibid., 220) has led to recent behavioural policies in health promotion and has tended to restrict the degree of social change. In the next section, health promotion's 'built-in tension that sometimes degenerates into a full-blown "paradigm war"' (Van Den Broucke 2014, 597) will be revisited with regard to its policy implications.

Comprehensive Concepts, Unbalanced Policies: The Mismatch Between Theory and Practice in Health Promotion

In the face of the ideological 'chasm' (Baum and Fisher 2014, 214) between advocates of different health promotion concepts, it is worth remembering that health promotion, or at least its recent history, has been based on a common conviction: 'Health is made outside the health care sector' (de Leeuw and Clavier 2011, ii237). Admittedly, even by the end of the nineteenth century, major public health achievements such as clean drinking water, sanitation facilities and workplace safety (Eyler and Brownson 2016) had been achieved through a broad suite of public policies not limited to health policy as such. After the Second World War, as national welfare systems were established and the 'healthcare state' came into being (Moran 1999), health maintenance became a professionalised and sectoralised affair. This meant that health policy was, in the main, limited to ensuring citizens' access to medical care in the case of illness, following a rationale of cure rather than prevention. Against this backdrop, new perspectives on health such as the *Lalonde Report* (1974) and Nancy Milio's (1981) famous book *Promoting Health through Public Policy* were ground-breaking. These pioneers of comprehensive health promotion concepts changed the underlying assumptions of health policies by putting 'health in the driving seat of social change' (Klein and Marmor 2012b, 506).

A New perspective on the Health of Canadians, a report commissioned by the then Canadian federal health (and former finance) minister Marc Lalonde (for detailed information on the making of the report, see McKay 2000), inspired other blueprints for health policymaking beyond the healthcare sector. Proposing an innovative health-field concept that consists of four health-affecting elements—human biology, environment, lifestyle and healthcare organisation—Lalonde's report provided 'a sort of map of the health territory' (Lalonde 1974, 31). Milio built on Lalonde's change of perspective concerning the nature of health by systematising the conditions for a more comprehensive approach, which was later labelled 'healthy public policy' (de Leeuw and Clavier 2011). Making the argument for cross-sectorial cooperation (in today's terms *Health-in-all-policies* approaches), Milio focused more specifically on the structural dimensions of promoting public health than Lalonde's conceptual ideas on the interplay between health determinants, and 'expounded a strategy rather than a program' (Klein and Marmor 2012b, 505). In retrospect, we can say that the Lalonde Report and Milio's book triggered a process that led to lasting changes in the underlying assumptions surrounding health. Both authors set the scene for a more holistic perspective on health (rather than healthcare), which culminated a few years later in the declaration of the Ottawa Charter (WHO 1986). The latter defined health promotion explicitly as a comprehensive *social and political* 'process of enabling people to increase control over, and improve their health (Nutbeam 1998, 351). Ideally, this vision is realised through a 'healthy public policy' (de Leeuw and Clavier 2011) based on 'enabling, mediating and advocating', as Kökény (2011) reminded us on the occasion of the 25th anniversary of the charter.

Problematically, at the level of policy implementation, policymakers have turned health promoters' carefully formulated *both-and* assumptions on health determinants and how to influence them into *either-or* decisions. In practice, policymakers have cherry-picked single recommendations (usually involving lifestyle aspects) while neglecting the overall thrust of health promotion concepts. Thus, in line with the normative aetiology outlined previously, health promotion policies that involve action at the level of individual behaviour have vastly outnumbered those that seek to change the structures and contexts within which individual health behaviour occurs (Baum 2015, 519–20). Moreover, as '[h]ealth translates into a product that can be bought on the market' (Kickbusch 2007, 152), new inroads for behavioural health promotion have emerged that turn healthy lifestyles into choices to be taken by health consumers.

On the other hand, mounting evidence concerning the impact of the social determinants of health (SDH) on health equity (Marmot 2005) has led to the foundation of a standing working unit on SDH by the WHO in 2008. So far, however, the imbalance in health promotion strategies pursued through public policy varies by country and over time. Almost instinctively, health policymakers' have chosen to tackle bad lifestyles (i.e. eating an unhealthy diet, taking insufficient exercise, excessive drinking and smoking) rather than bad social conditions (i.e. poor housing, unemployment, inequality) as the starting point for policy interventions. Even cherished community-based approaches, such as the former Finnish *North Karelia Program* to prevent coronary heart diseases and its successors (Puska 2008), are usually based on 'behavioural change theories' (Baum 2015, 509). Despite applying a comprehensive view of people's needs and fostering close cooperation with local stakeholders (including, in some cases, the food industry, supermarkets and the media), those programmes have to be carefully distinguished from broad health policies that, at least in theory, could question 'the power and influence of societal sectors to shape public policy' (Raphael 2014, 383).

It is only recently that the public health community (i.e. its academic and front-line pioneers) has started to analyse the reasons why the discipline 'has failed to enable, mediate and advocate for policy and political change' (de Leeuw and Clavier 2011, ii243). Explanations for this collective shortcoming include the rather naïve belief that scientific evidence on the SDH inevitably translates into policy (Baum and Fisher 2014), but also health promoters' 'neglect of politics, power and ideology' (Raphael

2014, 381) and/or their reluctance to engage in the tedious political arguments around policymaking in health promotion (ibid.). Against this backdrop, new policies in behavioural health promotion, most notably based on *nudges*, have become increasingly prominent. The subsequent section will turn to the question of how this 'behavioural turn' (Crawshaw 2013) may once again alter the underlying assumptions in policymaking for health promotion.

Nudge-Based Health Promotion: Game Changer or More of the Same?

In the face of a steep rise in the incidence of NCDs, the need for lifestyle changes can hardly be denied. Despite the tremendous impact of health-endangering environments such as *food deserts* on individual health behaviour, it is still individuals' co-responsibility to alter their own eating and exercise habits in order to improve their health. Due to its direct impact on individuals' health, which unlike the impact of social determinants is not abstract and can be experienced directly, 'behaviour does remain a critical determinant of health' (Van Den Broucke 2014, 597). At this point, behavioural public policies, mainly equated with the popular concept of 'nudges' (Thaler and Sunstein 2008; see also Chap. 3 of this volume), have raised hopes of new ways to improve public health. Essentially, nudging is both an old and a new strategy in health promotion: on the one hand, it builds on risk perception research and risk communication (Rudisill 2012), behavioural economics (Kahneman 2011) and social marketing (Crawshaw 2013), which have been components of health promotion policies for a long time. On the other hand, nudging is clearly new, in that it makes systematic use of evidence-based insights on human behaviour, which is evaluated through randomised control trials (John 2017). The latter provides *choice architects* in public policymaking with 'politico-epistemic authority' (Strassheim and Korinek 2016, 121). Applying this authority allows *health nudgers*, it is argued, to bypass the longstanding ideological cleavage between behavioural-focused and SDH-related policy approaches. In fact, at first glance 'nudging health' (Cohen et al. 2016) appears to be a reasonable middle ground that claims to innovatively address both the behavioural and socio-environmental dimensions of health promotion.

Based on the assumption that 'our choices are constantly at the behest of a myriad of influences' (Quigley 2013, 601), nudging systematically utilises these influences by reshaping the interplay between the environment and individual behaviour. Society's 'overall health picture' (ibid., 605), it is assumed, consists of countless health-affecting choice architectures such as the design of the built environment, how food is presented in shops or the availability of walking paths. Because, as is repeatedly stressed by Sunstein (e.g. 2014), choice architectures are *inevitable* and exist '[p]rior to any new policy' (Quigley 2013, 603), redesigning them is a key form of leverage in health promotion. Nudges take a wide range of forms, and relate to issues such as people's walking routines, smoking, drinking, eating and food-buying habits and the enhancement of public safety (OECD 2017). However, do the underlying assumptions of nudge policies differ from those of previous health promotion policies? And are they able to bridge the ideologically charged division lines that separate the various political camps in health promotion?

An evaluation of health nudges against the dimensions of policymakers' underlying assumptions concerning health promotion, as described above, produces a mixed picture. Firstly, by seeking behavioural change—the key rationale for health nudges—these policies are unambiguously 'based on an individual-level, psychological paradigm' (Spotswood and Marsh 2016, 284). However, in order to achieve healthier behaviours, choice architects reshape the contexts in which people are making their lifestyle choices. Hence, encouraging the use of stairs over elevators is a common health nudge that seeks to 'deconvenience people's life' (Carter 2015, 379). Significantly, nudgers assume that individual health represents people's major interest (White 2016) and therefore justifies behavioural intervention, whereas other human interests such as leisure and comfort are suspected of routinely undermining health's supremacy.

With regard to the second feature—the assumed causes of disease and, emanating from them, policymakers' prioritisation of health promotion policies—it is easier to classify nudging. Unequivocally, behavioural change policies focus exclusively on lifestyle risks and personal responsibility for presumably irrational behaviours on the part of individuals. Moreover, as Kelly (2016, 11) notes, those policies are 'never very far away from political and ideological beliefs about how people *ought* to be'. In this sense, nudge tactics correlate with the assumption that healthy lifestyles—strictly understood as being slim, active and drug-free—represent a universal ideal that is applicable to everyone and that can be achieved through 'prefabricated choice environments' (Leggett 2014, 13). Classified according to Kühn's normative aetiology, current nudge-based polices are very likely to be selected by health policymakers because they do not fundamentally seek to challenge environmental factors, social conditions or power relations, but concentrate 'narrowly on the choices made by individuals' (Owens and Cribb 2013, 268). Thus, far from being a game changer, today's light-touch, low-cost health nudges, fit almost seamlessly into the existing portfolio of health promotion policies 'where lifestyle health interventionism is already well established as the norm' (Burgess 2012, 16).

Moreover, like any other policy, nudging must be assessed within the spirit of the time and the political context in which it is applied. Steering people gently towards healthier choices is not an apolitical or neutral practice, even if it may appear to be. It is no coincidence that the mushrooming of nudge units across the globe is occurring in a social-political climate marked 'by citizen disillusionment with "politics as usual" and austerity' (Farrell 2017). Viewed in this way, behavioural policymaking in health promotion would seem to be a pragmatic 'way of dealing with the problematic consequences of neoliberalism' (Jones et al. 2013, 164) which have led to 'new social risks' (Bonoli 2005) such as precarious living conditions and scaled-back social security systems. For citizens, the underlying message that emanates from policymakers' appetite for health nudges sounds rather familiar: *there is no alternative* to behavioural change. These policies appear to be indispensable if lifestyle-driven diseases, which are associated with substantial costs, are to be avoided on a large scale. Framed in this manner, it is unsurprising that nudge tactics do not represent a greater challenge to what Raphael (2014) refers to as 'the raw politics behind opposition to healthy public policy', that is, the power of political forces and corporate actors that prevent societal and systemic change.

However, while recent behavioural policies are more likely to confirm rather than challenge the dominant assumptions in health policymaking, this does not mean that behavioural insights cannot be used to improve future health promotion policies. As Hallsworth et al. (2016, 12) note: '[I]t is clear that the full potential of a behavioral insights approach is yet to be realised – particularly in health'. For example, integrated policies that innovatively combine individual and societal interventions could benefit from behavioural insights. I will turn to this possibility in the next section.

Beyond Nudging: Is There a Role for Behavioural Insights in Health Promotion?

It should be clear by now that policymaking in health promotion has an 'obvious normative component' (Klein and Marmor 2012a, 2). Health policymakers draw from a limited reservoir of assumptions of what causes health and illness. Accordingly, health challenges such as NCDs seem almost exclusively to result from errant individuals 'struggling with their habits and willpower and self-regulation' (Spotswood and Marsh 2016, 284). It does not require a great deal of analytical acumen to realise that such a policy narrative is inadequate and simplistic, particularly in the face of wicked problems such as obesity. Given the wealth of studies that have revealed the complex interrelations between social determinants and people's eating behaviours (e.g. Bryant et al. 2015) and the ambitious concepts designed to address this nexus (Clavier and de Leeuw 2013), behavioural change theories appear ideologically motivated (Medvedyuk et al. 2017). On the contrary, it is argued, in order to be effective, health promotion policies require exactly the opposite: maximum independence and impartiality in relation to the choice of policy approaches and instruments (Van Den Broucke 2014). If they are understood as one (but not necessarily the primary) feature within a comprehensive and integrated approach, behavioural insights could well contribute to the overall success of health promotion policies. According to its recent reports, this view is increasingly shared by the UK Behavioural Insights Team (BIT) (Hallsworth et al. 2016; Halpern 2016).

A first step in this direction would be to widen the knowledge base that policymakers are drawing from when designing health promotion schemes. Such an 'expansion in the nature of evidence' (Spotswood and Marsh 2016, 290) is fundamental for concepts that seek to combine structural and individual measures of health promotion. Quantified insights into human behaviour, as produced by randomised controlled trials (RCTs), disguise the unquantifiable and contextual dimensions of unhealthy behaviours. Taking obesity as an example, these contextual dimensions concern the social settings, structures and interdependencies that obese people are confined to in their daily-lives. Evidence from RCTs, e.g. on the impact of smarter lunchrooms (Wansink 2016), is of little value if lunchroom visitors (e.g. students or employees) are simultaneously living in *food deserts* which reinforce rather than reduce poor dietary habits. Instead, obesity prevention requires a precise idea of the specific *flavour* of local settings, for example, on the particularities of food supply in local neighbourhoods and people's patterns of consumption. This information, which is localised by definition, can only be gathered through qualitative research (Spotswood and Marsh 2016) such as interviews and focus groups. In short, policymakers' assumptive worlds have to be nourished by a thick, real-world understanding of people's habits and lifestyles. As such, embedded social beings rather than anonymous study participants are the appropriate reference points for policymaking.

Secondly, the application of behavioural interventions in health policymaking must be reconceptualised. The crucial question is where (in which cases?) and when (within the policy process) policymakers should make use of behavioural insights. Reduced to its essence, behavioural policies are understood as 'interventions with a more realistic, and proven, understanding of human behaviour' (OECD 2017, 48). However, probably due to the discourse on bad lifestyles and individual responsibility for maintaining health, behavioural policies are too often equated with errant citizens who are prone to correction through nudging. However, Hallsworth et al. (2016, 12) claim that, in reality, 'behavioral insights should be seen as an approach to policymaking as a whole' which is applicable to every group of actors and at every stage of the health policy cycle (OECD 2017, 53). What is needed is a shift from nudging individual health at the level of policy implementation to the application of behavioural insights in the design of health promotion policies. With regard to 'healthy public policies' (de Leeuw and Clavier 2011), as-yet unfinished business such as cross-sectorial coordination and interprofessional cooperation could be re-examined through behavioural lenses. For example, administrative transparency and pro-cooperative behaviours, such as mutual exchange and shared decisions among stakeholders, could guide 'departments in applying cross-government agendas' (OECD 2017, 50). In this sense, a pivotal behavioural insight to be researched and utilised in policymaking concerns the determinants of stakeholders' behaviours which facilitate or impede collaboration in health promotion.

Thirdly, behavioural policies could be combined with participatory approaches to health promotion (John et al. 2009). Putting this suggestion into practice would elegantly circumvent a key criticism of behavioural policies—that is, elitism, which provokes the question *who nudges the nudgers?* Moreover, if Sunstein et al. (2017, 1–2) are right when they say that 'citizens generally approve of health and safety nudges' but 'do not approve of nudges that are perceived as having an illicit goal', a logical step would be to enhance the overall legitimacy of health nudges through deliberative procedures. Citizen juries, established to co-design health promotion strategies by applying local knowledge and experience, may opt to use health nudges as a component within a wider approach to health promotion. Citizen-approved nudges, for example, those that enhance neighbourhood walkability or access to nutritious food, would 'dispel any suspicion of manipulation or "tricking" citizens' (OECD 2017, 55) and may lead to better policy results. If deliberatively designed, health nudges are not restricted to the normative expectations of policymakers on how supposedly *ordinary* people should behave. On the contrary, they are examples of 'self-initiated efforts to improve [people's] decision-making' (White 2016, 31) in health-related situations.

To sum up, health promotion policies ought to be enhanced with pluralistic evidence, which includes but is not limited to behavioural insights, regarding what works in different settings. The as-yet untapped potential of behavioural insights includes the 'early design of policies' (OECD 2017, 53), that is, the setting up of a wide-ranging agenda for health promotion. In addition, health nudges, if approved and co-designed by citizens, could be a valuable component rather than a substitute for setting-based approaches to health promotion.

Some Final Remarks

There is little doubt that behavioural insights can 'offer new solutions to policy problems' (Hallsworth et al. 2016). If interpreted broadly, behaviourally informed policies could shake up and revitalise locked patterns in health promotion. However, to return to the global obesity crisis described at the beginning of the chapter, which underlying assumptions future policy interventions should be based on remains a point for debate. Is it wise to put all our faith in behavioural insights in the face of a large-scale epidemic such as obesity? In this respect, the results of *Victoria's Citizens' Jury on Obesity*[1] are extremely thought-provoking: established to propose *asks* (i.e. policy solutions) regarding how to combat obesity in this state in south-eastern Australia, the jury strongly emphasised the need for regulatory government interventions (Farrell 2017). According to the

[1] The around 100-member jury of 'everyday Victorians' was an initiative of *VicHealth* with support by *newDemocracy Foundation*. The jury run over a period of six weeks (Halpern 2016, 48).

jury, obesity prevention requires, above all, a ban on junk food and the marketing of soft drinks to children, a 20% on sugar-sweetened beverages and mandated discounts on healthy food for people living on lower incomes (VicHealth 2015). Remarkably, in the jury's final report, the term *behaviour* occurs just three times—in relation to increased government funding for skills-based learning programmes as well as improved access to health counselling for obese people (ibid.). Despite—or perhaps precisely because of—the constant political focus on individual lifestyles, the residents of Victoria seem to take an unbiased view of the range of policy actions that could be taken to promote public health. Significantly, they clearly prioritise structural changes within the social environments that shape health behaviours. Accordingly, subsidising citizens to buy healthier food is assumed to be a more effective approach than nudging them to eat healthily. If a citizen's jury initiated by an agency that is collaborating closely with BITs (Halpern 2016) attaches so little importance to behavioural policies, what does this tell us?

Despite people's general sympathy with health nudges (Sunstein et al. 2017) there seem to be concerns about whether the approach is always the most appropriate, especially if up-stream policies that regulate the health-affecting actions of corporate actors are insufficiently addressed by governments. With regard to complex issues such as obesity, regulative policies are necessary in order to protect people and enable them to maintain a balanced diet. In this respect, future lessons could be learned from tobacco prevention policies. In that area, it is considered proven that a combination of tax and price policies (Chaloupka et al. 2011) and the strict regulation of advertisement has successfully reduced tobacco use, accompanied by education, communication and public awareness strategies. A similar policy mix is required to tackle obesity. A first step would be, for example, the adoption of a uniform food traffic light and intelligent calorie-labelling system.[2] Labelling food in a way that shows its effects on health combines regulatory intervention (rating food using traffic light colours) with behavioural insights (people's choices are influenced by sub-conscious cues such as colours). Hence, a food traffic light system would represent a classic nudge, though one that would require state regulation to put in place. So far, within the European Union, massive resistance from food industry lobbyists has prevented any such regulation (Dionigi 2017,

[2] Accordingly, very fat or salty foods are labelled with a red traffic light, while healthy food such as fruit and vegetables are labelled with a green traffic light.

84–6). However, the current burden of NCDs is simply too heavy to rely one-sidedly on behavioural health policies as substitutes for more fundamental societal interventions. Finally, it is worth pondering which policy solutions might have been recommended by health promotion pioneers such as Lalonde and Milio. If we may be so bold, it is hard to believe that they would be jumping on the bandwagon and arguing that nudging behavioural change is a silver bullet in the fight against lifestyle diseases.

References

Baum, F. (2015). *The new public health*. Oxford: Oxford University Press.

Baum, F., & Fisher, M. (2014). Why behavioural health promotion endures despite its failure to reduce health inequities. *Sociology of Health & Illness, 36*(2), 213–225.

Bonoli, G. (2005). The politics of the new social policies: Providing coverage against new social risks in mature welfare states. *Policy and Politics, 33*(3), 431–449.

Bryant, P. H., Hess, A., & Bowen, B. G. (2015). Social determinants of health related to obesity. *The Journal for Nurse Practitioners, 11*(2), 220–225.

Burgess, A. (2012). Nudging' healthy lifestyles: The UK experiments with the behavioural alternative to regulation and the market. *European Journal of Risk Regulation, 1*, 3–16.

Cairney, P., & Oliver, K. (2017). Evidence-based policymaking is not like evidence-based medicine, so how far should you go to bridge the divide between evidence and policy? *Health Research Policy and Systems, 15*(1), 35.

Carpenter, D. (2012). Is health politics different? *Annual Review of Political Science, 15*(1), 287–311.

Carter, E. D. (2015). Making the blue zones: Neoliberalism and nudges in public health promotion. *Social Science and Medicine, 133*(2015), 374–382.

Chaloupka, F. J., Straif, K., & Leon, M. E. (2011). Effectiveness of tax and price policies in tobacco control. *Tobacco Control, 2011*(20), 235–238.

Clavier, C., & de Leeuw, E. (2013). *Health promotion and the policy process*. Oxford: Oxford University Press.

Cohen, G. I., Lynch, H. F., & Robertson, C. T. (2016). *Nudging health: Health law and behavioral economics*. Baltimore: John Hopkins University Press.

Crawford, R. (1980). Healthism and the medicalization of everyday life. *International Journal of Health Services, 10*(3), 365–388.

Crawshaw, P. (2013). Public health policy and the behavioural turn: The case of social marketing. *Critical Social Policy, 33*(4), 616–637.

de Leeuw, E., & Clavier, C. (2011). Healthy public in all policies. *Health Promotion International, 26*, ii237. https://doi.org/10.1093/heapro/dar071.

Dionigi, M. K. (2017). *Lobbying in the European Parliament: The battle for influence*. London: Palgrave Macmillan.
Eyler, A. A., & Brownson, R. C. (2016). The power of policy to improve health. In A. A. Eyler, J. F. Chriqui, S. Moreland-Russell, & R. C. Brownson (Eds.), *Prevention, policy, and public health* (pp. 3–16). Oxford: Oxford University Press.
Farrell, A.-M. (2017, June 27). *The politics of behavioural policymaking in health promotion: Exploring recent developments in Australia*. Presentation held at the 3rd international conference on public policy (ICPP), Singapore.
Hallsworth, M., Snijders, V., Burd, H., Prestt, J., Judah, G., Huf, S., & Halpern, D. (2016). *Applying behavioural insights. Simple ways to improve health outcomes*. Doha: World Innovation Summit for Health.
Halpern, D. (2016). *Behavioural insights and healthier lives*. Melbourne: Victorian Health Promotion Foundation.
John, P. (2017). Behavioural science, randomised evaluations and the transformation of public policy. The case of the UK government. In J. Pykett, R. Jones, & M. Whitehead (Eds.), *Psychological governance and public policy: Governing the mind, brain and behaviour* (pp. 136–152). London/New York: Routledge.
John, P., Smith, G., & Stroker, G. (2009). Nudge nudge, think think: Two strategies of changing civic behaviour. *The Political Quarterly, 80*(3), 361–370.
Jones, R., Pykett, J., & Whitehead, M. (2013). Psychological governance and behaviour change. *Policy & Politics, 41*(2), 159–182.
Kahneman, D. (2011). *Thinking, fast and slow*. London: Penguin Books.
Kelly, M. P. (2016). The politics of behaviour change. In F. Spotswood (Ed.), *Beyond Behaviour Change. Key issues, interdisciplinary approaches and future directions* (pp. 11–26). Bristol: Policy Press.
Kickbusch, I. (2007). Health governance: The health society. In D. V. McQueen, I. Kickbusch, & L. Potvin (Eds.), *Health and modernity: The role of theory in health promotion* (pp. 144–161). Berlin: Springer.
Klein, R., & Marmor, T. (2012a). Politics and policy analysis: Fundamentals. In T. Marmor & R. Klein (Eds.), *Politics, health and health care* (pp. 1–21). New Haven/London: Yale University Press.
Klein, R., & Marmor, T. (2012b). New paradigms: Health care to population health. In T. Marmor & R. Klein (Eds.), *Politics, health and health care* (pp. 504–506). New Haven/London: Yale University Press.
Kökény, M. (2011). Ottawa revisited: 'Enable, mediate and advocate'. *Health Promotion International, 26*(S2), ii180–ii182.
Kühn, H. (1993). *Healthismus: Eine Analyse der Präventionspolitik und Gesundheitsförderung in den U.S.A.* Berlin: edition sigma.
Lalonde, M. (1974). *A new perspective on the health of Canadians*. Ottawa: Government of Canada.
Leggett, W. (2014). The politics of behaviour change: Nudge, neoliberalism and the state. *Policy & Politics, 42*(1), 3–19.

Lemke, T. (2013). *Perspectives on genetic discrimination*. New York: Routledge.
Marmot, M. (2005). Social determinants of health inequalities. *Lancet, 365*(9464), 1099–1104.
McKay, L. (2000). *Making the lalinde report. Towards a new perspective on health project*, Health Network, CPRN (Background Paper). Retrieved May 18, 2018 from http://epe.lac-bac.gc.ca/100/200/300/cdn_policy_research_net/making_lalonde/bmlr_e.pdf.
Medvedyuk, S., Ahmednur, A., & Raphael, D. (2017). Ideology, obesity and the social determinants of health: A critical analysis of the obesity and health relationship. *Critical Public Health*. doi:https://doi.org/10.1080/09581596.2017.1356910.
Milio, N. (1981). *Promoting health through public policy*. Philadelphia: F.A. Davis Company.
Moran, M. (1999). *Governing the health care state. A comparative study of the United Kingdom, the United States and Germany*. Manchester: Manchester University Press.
Nutbeam, D. (1998). Health promotion glossary. *Health Promotion International, 13*(4), 349–364.
OECD. (2017). *Behavioural insights and public policy: Lessons from around the world*. Paris: OECD Publishing.
Owens, J., & Cribb, A. (2013). Beyond choice and individualism: Understanding autonomy for public health ethics. *Public Health Ethics, 6*(3), 262–271.
Peters, B. G., & Zittoun, P. (2016). Introduction. In B. G. Peters & P. Zittoun (Eds.), *Contemporary approaches to public policy* (pp. 1–14). London: Palgrave Macmillan.
Puska, P. (2008). The North Karelia project: 30 years successfully preventing chronic diseases. *Diabetes Voice, 53*(Special issue), 26–29.
Quigley, M. (2013). Nudging for health: On public policy and designing choice architecture. *Medical Law Review, 21*(2013), 588–621.
Raphael, D. (2011). A discourse analysis of the social determinants of health. *Critical Public Health, 21*(2), 221–236.
Raphael, D. (2014). Beyond policy analysis: The raw politics behind opposition to healthy public policy. *Health Promotion International, 30*(2), 380–396.
Rudisill, C. (2012). Risk research and health-related behaviours. In A. McGuire & L. Costa-Font (Eds.), *The LSE companion to health policy* (pp. 297–313). Cheltenham/Northampton: Edward Elgar.
Spotswood, F. (2016). Introduction. In F. Spotswood (Ed.), *Beyond behaviour change. Key issues, interdisciplinary approaches and future directions* (pp. 1–8). Bristol: Policy Press.
Spotswood, F., & Marsh, A. (2016). Conclusion: What is the future of 'behaviour change'? In F. Spotswood (Ed.), *Beyond behaviour change. Key issues, interdisciplinary approaches and future directions* (pp. 283–298). Bristol: Policy Press.

Strassheim, H., & Korinek, R.-L. (2016). Cultivating 'nudge': Behavioural governance in the UK. In J. P. Voß & R. Freeman (Eds.), *Knowing governance. The epistemic construction of political order* (pp. 107–126). New York: Palgrave Macmillan.

Sunstein, C. (2014). *Why nudge? The politics of libertarian paternalism.* New Haven/London: Yale University Press.

Sunstein, C. R., Reisch, L. A., & Rauber, J. (2017). A worldwide consensus on nudging? Not quite, but almost. *Regulation & Governance, 12*, 3. https://doi.org/10.1111/rego.12161.

Thaler, R., & Sunstein, C. (2008). *Nudge: Improving decisions about health, wealth and happiness.* New York: Penguin Books.

Van Den Broucke, S. (2014). Needs, norms and nudges: The place of behaviour change in health promotion (editorial). *Health Promotion International, 29*(4), 597–600.

VicHealth. (2015). *Citizen's Jury on Obesity*, online available via https://www.vichealth.vic.gov.au/programs-and-projects/victorias-citizens-jury-on-obesity. 17 Dec 2017.

Wansink, B. (2016). Slim by design: Moving from Can't to CAN. In C. A. Roberto & I. Kawachi (Eds.), *Behavioral economics and public health* (pp. 237–264). Oxford: Oxford University Press.

White, M. D. (2016). Bad medicine: Does the unique nature of healthcare decisions justify nudges? In G. I. Cohen, H. F. Lynch, & C. T. Robertson (Eds.), *Nudging health: Health law and behavioral economics* (pp. 72–82). Baltimore: John Hopkins University Press.

WHO. (1986). *Ottawa charter for health promotion.* Retrieved December 29, 2017 from http://www.euro.who.int/__data/assets/pdf_file/0004/129532/Ottawa_Charter.pdf?ua=1.

WHO. (2017). *Obesity and overweight.* Fact sheet. Retrieved December 29, 2017 from http://www.who.int/mediacentre/factsheets/fs311/en/.

CHAPTER 3

Approaches and Instruments in Health Promotion and the Prevention of Diseases

Kathrin Loer

Abstract Policy instruments do not only express how policymakers expect citizens or corporate actors to behave. The implementation of policy instruments also affects citizens and corporate actors directly and indirectly. The chapter brings together public health discourse, concepts and insights from political science on policy instruments. It enhances the instrument typology in order to understand the influence of behavioural insights on policy instruments. The chapter explains how "classical" instruments can be informed by behavioural science and under which circumstances behavioural insights offer a chance to change both the social environment and the individual behaviour that occurs in that environment, by focusing on building a choice architecture that promotes healthier behaviours.

Keywords Policy instruments • Behavioural insights • Public health • Choice architecture

K. Loer (✉)
FernUniversität in Hagen, Hagen, Germany
e-mail: kathrin.loer@fernuni-hagen.de

B. Ewert, K. Loer (eds.), *Behavioural Policies for Health Promotion and Disease Prevention*, Palgrave Studies in Public Health Policy Research, https://doi.org/10.1007/978-3-319-98316-5_3

Introduction

Policy instruments do not only express how policymakers expect citizens or corporate actors to behave. The implementation of policy instruments also affects citizens and corporate actors directly and indirectly. Imagine a situation in which a specific substance, which people regularly consume and producers earn money from, was prohibited. Both producers and consumers would be affected by political processes, since policymakers decide on the type of instrument or mix of instruments that is applied, the degree of coerciveness and the scope of application. These decisions typically follow various forms of bargaining between policymakers and stakeholders (cp. Chap. 5). That said, it is patently obvious that the issue of "policy instruments" is a core topic in political science and can be applied to several areas of policymaking. But policy instruments play a particularly important role in public health. Promoting public health and reducing ill health require appropriate strategies. The constituent elements of those strategies are instruments, even though public health literature often refers to "policies" when instruments are meant. There is a need to bring together public health discourse and concepts and insights from political science on policy instruments. This chapter will do exactly this, merging the instrument discourse that is used in political science with the broad spectrum of issues and concepts used in public health, which have changed over time.

In addition to merging the discourses of public health and political science, it would also be useful to integrate ideas and concepts from behavioural sciences when discussing policy instruments. The explosive growth in "nudges" (Thaler and Sunstein 2008) and other tools that emanate from behavioural research is inspiring the debate on public health, but it is also giving rise to controversies and misunderstandings. This chapter will therefore present an idea of how to deal with new forms of policymaking/new policies that are based (mainly) on behavioural sciences. This relates closely to Ewert's chapter on underlying assumptions (Chap. 2), which are important to understanding the context of policymaking in public health. But instruments also relate directly to the subsequent chapter on examples of policymaking (Chap. 4), since Pykett shows what kind of (behavioural) instruments are being implemented effectively in various countries. To understand which interests play a role when particular instruments are chosen, combined and applied, Loer and Strassheim's chapter (Chap. 5) provides further insights. All this can be better understood if we systematically distinguish the different types of instruments and reflect on the limits and conditions of their application.

Since instruments are closely linked to political issues or problem structures (cp. Introduction), a brief outline of issues in public health will first be provided. Public health research has shown how health was recognised and how this recognition changed over time. Although we can observe times of technology-based health perspectives and biomedical models of health (de Leeuw 2017, 330), there is also the idea of a "health society" and its characteristics explained from a sociological perspective (Kickbusch 2007). What we learn from this literature is that health is created in social and physical environments and "outside health sectors" (de Leeuw 2017, 330). This said, public health has to apply methods of political engagement across levels (de Leeuw 2017, 341).

Although modern public health would have to follow such ideas of cross-sectoral engagement, the policy debate is often narrowed to the following issues: (1) fighting communicable diseases (CDs), (2) developing population-based approaches to promoting health and preventing diseases and (3) providing medical services or personal health services in cases that are not covered by the national healthcare system (Asch et al. 2005, 533). While few changes have occurred in relation to the third mission[1] and this is closely linked to the specifics of national health systems, the first two missions depend on a range of factors. CDs have been the major challenge in the history of public health: improvements in sanitation and housing, cleanliness and (scientific) research on how to prevent epidemics (such as smallpox, diphtheria, malaria, leprosy, plague) remained on the agenda for centuries (Rosen 2015). Policymakers ensured the development of health infrastructure: hospitals emerged, and hygiene and sanitation standards were introduced and resulted in fewer infections and reductions in mortality (Evans et al. 1994, 10). The social and environmental determinants of health played a decisive role in maintaining people's health and were addressed. Public health measures often implied strict regulation (e.g. bans, legislative measures) but also information campaigns (e.g. to promote better hygiene standards). In the case of CDs, the political debate focused on the state's duties to protect citizens from the major threats that

[1] This can, of course, become more relevant in times when more people are (more or less suddenly) not covered by a national health service or insurance schemes (e.g. during an exceptional influx of refugees who are not automatically entitled for benefits).

emerged due to urbanisation and industrialisation. Although there are still lively debates on vaccination (e.g. Verweij and Houweling 2014) and on how to cope with epidemics (though less so in industrialised countries), CDs have largely been replaced by non-communicable diseases (NCDs) when it comes to the major health threats faced in developed countries (and, these days, in emerging countries too).

NCDs include a variety of "chronic conditions" that may to a greater or lesser extent be related to individual behaviours. Industrialisation led to a rise in chronic health conditions due to injuries sustained at work—whether due to poor working conditions and safety standards and/or personal negligence—or due to pollution (Milio 1981, 15). Crash-related morbidity resulting from cars and traffic accidents (including, e.g. cyclists) is a similar example. However, international health statistics and major national and international debates on public health reveal that policymakers tend to focus on NCDs that are associated with personal behaviour rather than social determinants: overeating, poor nutrition, alcohol consumption, smoking, drug use (Milio 1981, 16f.) are all major focus areas. Without deciding who is primarily responsible for the emergence of NCDs, we recognise that individual *and* social determinants are both relevant to health. However, public policies for health increasingly seem to demonstrate the interplay and complex tension between approaches and instruments that focus on individuals' behaviour, with interventions that focus on individuals, such as those that aim to facilitate healthier choices, getting the most attention, whereas societal interventions that focus on the social and environmental determinants of health (i.e. political, spatial and social factors that shape health and health behaviour) are often neglected. As Purnell et al. put it, the "policy agenda in this area remains underdeveloped" (Purnell et al. 2016). One reason for this could be the inherent dynamics of the policy-process, power relations and institutional dynamics or inertia. Before discussing these aspects and the dynamics of policy-processes and power relations (see the following chapters of this book), it is useful to explore the types of policy instruments that are relevant in public health.

Various dimensions play a role when examining instruments in policy-making: We shall consider a useful typology before becoming more specific. We shall conceptualise policy targets or addressees that are often overlooked in the debate on policy instruments. And we shall consider whether policy instruments should be classified as high or low population agency (see Chap. 1), which essentially corresponds to the degree of coerciveness that is involved. It is also useful to better consider the difference between policy targets. And finally, we will address the general questions of which instruments are applied and in which areas of public health, how specific instruments are used and how behavioural insights (can) change policy instruments in public health.

Typology of Instruments: What Does This Mean in Public Health?

Public health involves highly complex and wide-ranging issues (for an overview see Chap. 1) and policymakers can choose from a wide variety of options. But policymaking in public health is not only oriented towards specific solutions that need to be found for particular problems. This chapter is based on the assumption that there is neither a distinct problem-solution-nexus nor a strict correlation between issues/problems and policy instruments. It follows the idea of multiple streams (Kingdon 1995) which is already applied to public health policy (e.g. de Leeuw et al. 2016, de Leeuw 2017; in contrast to the—misleading—idea of a "policy-cycle", e.g. in Jann and Wegrich 2007). Which issues effectively make it onto the agenda will always depend heavily on which policy instruments are available, and vice versa, but institutions, actor's beliefs and interests and situational elements also play a major role (Böcher and Töller 2016). Even if pressure from civil society or exogeneous shocks to the policy network have an influence on agenda-setting the availability of policy instruments will be a determining factor. As such, choosing instruments is part of political processes which does not generally follow a functional concept of problem and solution. Additionally, we see changes over time, not only with regard to the issues that make it onto the agenda but also in terms of the instruments used.

Political scientists and legal scholars have developed a variety of policy instrument typologies. They range from those that are limited to three types (Lowi 1972) to typologies that comprise up to 40 or more instruments (e.g. Kirschen 1969). These typologies, some of them highly complex, are not likely to yield plausible and comprehensible analyses on how behavioural change is set in motion, however. Hitherto, the effect of behavioural insights has not been systematically integrated into the debate on policy instruments (for a first approach on instrument typology that integrates behavioural insights see Loer 2018). When arguing for a new heuristic for policy instruments, the principle of Occam's Razor shall serve as a guideline in order to keep this simple and limit the number of types of instruments. After comparing the wide range of typologies and distilling the pivotal ideas, this chapter will describe four distinct policy instrument types and explain their role in public health policymaking. The following section will provide a political science perspective on those instruments, introduce a typology of the four instruments as a basis and then proceed to show how behavioural insights affect these instruments.

Each instrument will briefly be discussed by answering the following questions: what is its main characteristic and what are its distinctive features? Can several tools be grouped together? Which underlying mechanisms can be identified in the instruments? What role does the state play when applying these instruments? What "limits and coins" (Hood 1983 introduced the terms categories for the instrument's limits and coins understood in a figurative sense as not only financial costs or expenses) can be expected with regard to the use of the respective instrument? An instrument's limit is reached when the negative effects of its use outweigh its expected advantages. The "coins" of an instrument are the constraints that policymakers have to consider when using an instrument, and relate to the costs of the instrument (and not only in financial terms).

Generally speaking, political scientists understand instruments as "a set of techniques by which governmental authorities wield their power in attempting to ensure support and effect (or prevent) social change" (Vedung 2003, 21). Whether or not this goal can be achieved depends on the effectiveness of the instrument, which in turn relates to the fit between the character of the instrument and its mechanisms, provided that the addressee is responsive to these characteristics—a highly relevant factor particularly in public health.

A better understanding of these aspects will help to analyse instruments and instrument mixes better, and to explain their shortcomings. Furthermore, a better understanding of instruments should include an answer to the question of how behavioural insights are applied in policymaking and how they may affect instruments. This questions follows an initial classification of "nudges" as being a "complement to the traditional policy instruments" or their combination (e.g. Lehner et al. 2015, 166).[2] This is not inconsistent with Sunstein's idea that "Nudges are private or public initiatives that steer people in particular directions but that also

[2] Although Lehner et al. (2015) use the term "complement", they present different varieties of "nudge mechanisms" understood as an addition to traditional policy tools, see p. 168.

allow them to go their own way" (Sunstein 2017). However, political science researchers have yet to demonstrate how nudges can be conceptualised in concrete terms and align them with the classical instrument typologies of political science.

Most of the prevailing instrument typologies in political sciences begin with "control" (or command and control) and can be distinguished from "distribution" (or "re-distribution") instruments. Theodore Lowi's lean and elegant typology laid the groundwork for all subsequent research. He identifies several classifications of instruments: distributive, redistributive, regulatory and constituent (Lowi 1972). A survey of the broad literature on instruments and the tools of government basically repeats and confirms Lowi's classification but adds an important additional category: "authority", "incentive", "capacity" and (additionally) "organisation". The inclusion of this extra category not only means incorporating the extensive literature that shows how important and relevant this instrument is (e.g. Böcher 2012), but it also adds a fourth dimension to the triad that is sufficiently different from the three instruments already mentioned and plays a major role in public health and behavioural insights.

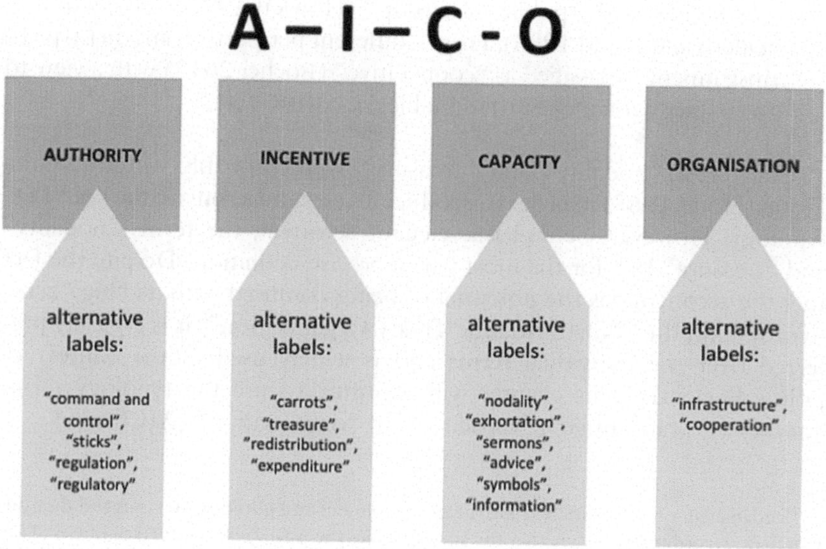

Fig. 3.1 Instruments—Varieties of labelling. (Illustration based on literature dealing with policy instruments)

Despite some semantic differences, the typological terms used by scholars over the last 30 years are surprisingly similar. The literature reveals several terms used to classify these four types of instrument:

- authoritative instruments such as "command and control" are known as **authority** (Schneider and Ingram 1990; C. C. Hood 1983) but also as "sticks" (Vedung 2003) or regulatory/regulation (e.g. Böcher 2012);
- incentivising instruments are classified as treasure (C. C. Hood 1983), **incentive** (Schneider and Ingram 1990), carrots (Vedung 2003), economic instruments (Böcher 2012) or expenditure (Howlett 1991);
- instruments that focus on capacity-building are referred to as: nodality (Hood 1983), **capacity** (Schneider and Ingram 1990), sermons (Vedung 2003), persuasive instruments (Böcher 2012), exhortation (Howlett 1991);
- cooperative and organisational instruments fall into a broader category: **organisation** is presented as a distinct category meaning bureaucratic administration or running public enterprises. Howlett follows a similar idea with "public ownership" (Howlett 1991 in adaptation of Doern and Phidd 1983). From a different perspective, another type of instrument is classified as "cooperative" (Böcher 2012) with a view to voluntary agreements, round tables, mediation etc.

The terms "nodality" and "treasure" were probably introduced by Hood (Hood 1983) in order to produce an elegant acronym: the "NATO" typology. However, behind this elegant acronym, the terms "nodality" and "treasure" lack for the most part a precise definition. Despite the fact that the acronym has the potential of being confused with its "big" acronym sibling, the "North Atlantic Treaty Organization", it is typically preferred over the individual terms and is widely used in the context of political science. This chapter will continue to use the typology terms "**a**uthority", "**i**ncentive", "**c**apacity" and "**o**rganisation" (AICO).[3]

[3] Jordan et al. propose different instrument typologies and government types and they differentiate according to (a) whether the state specifies the goal to be achieved or not, and (b) whether the state specifies how the goal is to be achieved (Jordan et al. 2005). Although this matrix (four fields) could be helpful for specific analysis it mixes different types of instruments and could lead to some confusion.

To better understand the characteristics of each instrument, the following paragraphs will discuss the four types of instrument in the context of empirical examples from public health and, in a second step, will emphasise one specific example to be used when discussing behavioural insights later. Tobacco control is chosen as the specific empirical case: the goal of the policy is to respond to the political question of how best to reduce the use of tobacco in order to protect the individual's health and public health. There are five main reasons why the example of tobacco regulation is appropriate: (1) the use of instruments to regulate tobacco (production and use) has a long history; (2) the medical need to reduce individual's tobacco consumption in order to prevent certain diseases (e.g. cancer, cardio-vascular diseases, etc.) is no longer (politically) disputed; (3) tobacco is an issue for policymaking in many countries worldwide; (4) it has been targeted not only by governments but also by international and supranational organisations (the EU, WHO, etc.); and (5) different instruments were and are used in relation to tobacco regulation. This example could be transferred to other urgent issues in contemporary public health that relate to substances such as the overconsumption of sugar or alcohol, for example; however, it is necessary to recognise not only that each substance requires its own specific approach when it comes to the regulatory details, but also that the medical evidence of adverse health effects remains controversial, which has an impact on policymaking.

In the following section, each instrument discussed is conceptualised to serve as a distinct category of instrument. The description not only maps out the instrument's general characteristics, its limits and coins (i.e. the resources needed to implement the instrument), and its degree of coerciveness, but it also outlines the concept of the addressee in order to understand which mechanisms are triggered by the instrument. So far, the literature on instrument typologies does not systematically point out that the addressee is a relevant concept. Only Howlett suggests introducing what he calls "Target Behaviour Pre-Requisite" and presents four relevant aspects: willingness to (a) "be manipulated by force" (authority) or (b) "be manipulated by gain/losses" (incentive) or (c) "believe info" (information) or (d) "receive goods and services from government" (Howlett 2016, 17f.). The following section develops a similar idea but suggests a specific addressee concept, which is somewhat different from the "Target Behaviour Pre-Requisite".

Authority

The highest degree of coercion is achieved when authority is used, that is, when policymakers make decisions in a command-and-control manner. Prohibition or command (prescriptive rules) entail the severest intervention into the liberties of individual or corporate actors. Furthermore, there must be an effective system of observation and sanctioning in order to achieve a degree of effectiveness. If the addressee is convinced of the rules, he or she will most likely simply comply. But otherwise, deterrent sanctions are required to push him or her towards the intended behaviour. Although it is theoretically possible to fully prohibit the use of tobacco, the political limitations of prohibition are obvious when it comes to tobacco regulation. A clear distinction needs to be made between children, young people and adults. The prohibition of tobacco use for children and youth is generally non-controversial. The restrictions applied fairly recently on tobacco use in public places (such as bars and restaurants) have now been broadly accepted wherever introduced. Over the past 10–15 years, many countries have implemented tobacco restrictions, a trend that began in US states in the 1970s and 1980s. More extensive and coercive regulations, however, would seem politically risky due to the interests of both smokers, the tobacco industry (Brownell and Warner 2009; Nathanson 1999; Richardson 2015) and governments themselves (who benefit from tax revenues). The example of tobacco shows that regulation can be directed towards consumers or producers, but it requires a broad political and social consensus among voters, organised interests and market actors if it is to be accepted. If such a consensus is lacking, political actors would expect to be punished at the ballot box after introducing a total tobacco ban, for example. But, if accepted, the use of authority can lay the ground for a level playing field since the same rules are applied for all citizens or companies in a particular sector. It can be classified as a "low population agency" approach, but ultimately it is dependent on enough addressees (citizens) being willing to comply with the new rules. For this reason, interventions aimed at limiting the individual consumption of a particular product, or banning its consumption altogether, must always be considered carefully (for an overview of political discourse in this field see Brownell and Warner 2009; Nathanson 1999; Richardson 2015). Similar political effects can be observed when it comes to the strict(er) regulation of vaccinations, for example. An absolute safeguard against all infectious diseases for which there is a vaccine can only exist if the state introduces compulsory vaccinations and enforces this obligation to the best of its ability. At the same time, vaccinations affect individuals' fundamental right to physical integrity, i.e. the right to self-determination in matters relating to the body. This creates the need for state legitimation. However, the use of authority—if a decision to act is made—can be legitimised as the result of a democratic decision-making procedure. Theoretically, everyone can observe the political process. It is transparent and based on political discourse. When using the "authority" instrument, a distinct concept is adopted of the addressee who—for whatever reason—complies with the rules. Provided the addressee is compliant, the state will refrain from imposing sanctions.

Incentives

The introduction of taxes or subsidies is based on the assumption that economic incentives have a steering effect.[4] The same is supposed to be the case for non-economic incentives, that is, tools that enhance reputation, award prizes and awards and so on. The health damage caused by tobacco consumption and the associated costs may make it possible to justify taxing tobacco purchases in political rhetoric.[5] This distinct economic incentive has been used in many countries for years and is still strongly supported by the WHO as "the most effective approach to controlling the spread of tobacco use" (http://www.who.int/tobacco/economics/taxation/en/), and is part of the WHO Framework Convention on Tobacco Control (Article 6). If governments decide against prohibiting a particular product or substance, how can they achieve the goal of reducing its use (or other substances that are adverse to human health)? Governments can introduce a variety of economic incentives: taxes on products or production, minimum prices or incentives linked to the results of tobacco use: higher insurance rates for smokers, for example. All types of incentive, and especially the financial type, are based on the assumption of economic rationality and the addressee as a rational actor. The limits of

[4] During the 2000s, incentivizing instruments seem to have been the most important instruments used in policymaking—especially in the European Union. For an in-depth analysis see, among others, examples from environmental policy (Jordan et al. 2005; Knill and Lenschow 2005).

[5] Although one would expect to see a direct link between taxes and health costs, studies show that this direct link does not exist.

this instrument are obvious, however: if targeted taxation or other financial incentives are not high enough, the effect will be small; thus, subsidies, grants or financial support are literally the coin of this instrument since financial resources are needed. However, higher taxes can also be costly in political terms, as tax rates must remain reasonable. Taxes restrict the liberty of producers to fully exploit market demand and they limit the consumers' ability or propensity to consume a product, depending on their individual budget. The literal "coin" of this instrument is money, i.e. the use of taxes and subsidies. Taxes and subsidies are an institutionalisation of the political goal, and they are visible to consumers and producers. Similarly, as with "authority", the use of taxes—if chosen—derives its legitimacy from the political decision-making procedure and is based on a concrete and transparent political debate on the introduction of a tax, which is typically accompanied by media coverage. Economic incentives presume economic rationality in its purest form. Non-financial incentives are also based on the assumption that the addressee will follow a specific rationality: he or she prefers not to lose social reputation or will take the opportunity to enhance his or her reputation. If "incentives" are chosen as a policy instrument, political actors assume their addressees to be highly rational.

Capacity

Given the limitations of authority and incentives, governments would be sensible to use informational tools. Information is needed to convince people to change their habits or make the "right" lifestyle choices. Training, education and other provisions can ensure that individuals are in possession of all relevant information. It is generally assumed that people will make the best choices for themselves and their environment if they are well-informed. Obviously, governments have little to lose from a publicity campaign or other informational activities. The case of tobacco is a popular example of a capacity-building tool, but the use of these tools could easily be transferred to other substances or behavioural patterns (e.g. encouraging people to take more exercise). Governmental initiatives to inform and educate people start from the assumption that these initiatives are independent of economic interests and based on evidence from scientific studies, experts and so on. Therefore, the instrument of capacity-building takes its strength from the assumed neutrality, reputation and expertise of the state, which acts in an institutionalised manner and is transparent in its proceedings. However, such measures depend on consumers who understand the information provided and who translate that into actual behaviours. The basis of capacity-building and informational instruments is the conviction that the citizen as an addressee will act reasonably and, to a certain degree, intelligently. But it also requires the state to be recognised as credible. The case of tobacco case is well suited to an assessment of the effectiveness of capacity-building tools since although information campaigns now have a long history, people are still consuming tobacco. This is also the case when it comes to campaigns to promote physical activity, change people's eating habits or convince them to drink less alcohol. Even though people are (often) aware of the adverse health effects of their lifestyles and may even have considered quitting smoking, doing more exercise, changing their diet, or reducing their alcohol intake, they will not necessarily act accordingly and continue to have lifestyles that are sub-optimal in terms of health. However, capacity-building tools are generally accepted because they view citizens as responsible consumers. At the same time, however, this type of instrument challenges the consumer's weaknesses when it comes to established habits and practices. Like "authority" and "incentive", they are based on concrete and transparent communication: since this instrument is based on the addressee being in agreement with the information, it is also based on communication (Lascoumes and Le Galès 2007).

Organisation

The category of "organisation" covers various types of tools. At its least coercive, the state could initiate voluntary regulation, which means that organisations, associations or companies come together to agree on policies in a specific field. Policymakers sometimes coordinate voluntary agreements; these can often be classified as a way for non-state actors to prevent regulation or stricter regulation. Political scientists point to this phenomenon as a process that takes place in the "shadow of hierarchy" (for thorough studies in environmental policies and the specific case of pharmaceutical industries see Töller 2013, 2017). Other than that, slightly more state intervention can be observed in cases where the state initiates roundtables or other forms of cooperation between state and non-state actors. Similarly, civil society may be included and therefore be motivated to act in a specific way or to make the decisions that policymakers expect. A different version of organisational instruments is public ownership or public service delivery. Offering public infrastructure or services directly enables the state to influence the supply that people can consume, and thereby to structure the decision-making process. Organisation could be observed in cases of public ownership (i.e. state enterprises) which were traditionally used in a number of countries as a way of achieving various policy goals. In the case of alcohol, for example, state ownership was used (and is still the norm in Canada) as a way of complementing regulation with the goal of limiting consumption and/or restricting access by vulnerable groups such as young people. The case of the German tobacco sector involves a voluntary agreement whereby the industry has adopted voluntary agreements in order to prevent stricter advertising regulations or a complete ban on tobacco advertising. The case of tobacco shows that regulations on advertising and promotional campaigns are becoming ever more restrictive, mainly driven by the European Union, and organisational instruments are often a precursor to stricter regulations (authority and incentives). Sometimes, the same is true of initiatives for state-led committees, roundtables or panels: they can serve as a first step towards the use of one or more of the other instruments. In any case, it is the "organising state" that seeks to be less interventionist and promotes participation, in the expectation of cooperative addressees. With regard to these addressees, it is important to stress that they will only be cooperative if they recognise added value, for example, if they expect a reduction in transaction costs or if they see an opportunity to prevent stricter forms of regulation.

First Results

The case of tobacco shows that all four instruments are in use. With regard to other spheres of public health regulation, governments sometimes combine two or more instruments together closely in order to achieve their policy goals more effectively. But all these instruments, even when combined, have their limits and suffer from limited effectiveness. The fact that people are still addicted to smoking and young people are still taking up smoking shows that tobacco regulations have not been entirely effective. The picture becomes much more complicated when we broaden our perspective to include other substances and activities that have adverse health effects and are in some cases becoming major threats to public health: poor nutrition, sedentary behaviour, drug addiction, gambling and the like. Nevertheless, the examples have shown that the focus on the addressee is key.

Regardless of the concrete choice of instrument(s), all four types of instrument—authority, incentive, capacity and organisation—are based on the idea of a—more or less—rational addressee. Yet they do not incorporate ideas from behavioural sciences. The instruments also fail to incorporate aspects like social pressures or patterns as well as the non-cognitive dimensions of behaviour. What all the instruments have in common is that they are based on communicative acts and involve state institutions that can be observed by the public and, ultimately, held to account by democratic means. Thus, they stand for a specific kind of relationship between the state and its citizens: "A public policy instrument constitutes a device that is both technical and social, that organises specific social relations between the state and those it is addressed to, according to the representations and meanings it carries. It is a particular type of institution, a technical device with the generic purpose of carrying a concrete concept of the politics/society relationship and sustained by a concept of regulation" (Lascoumes and Le Galès 2007, 4). The citizen is the recipient of information (in its broadest sense, including information about a prohibition, an obligation, a tax, etc.) and the state provides tools in which rules equate to authority, taxes equate to incentives; campaigns equate to capacity; and infrastructure equates to organisation. The communicative act must be considered as the key when governments apply instruments—after all, they must communicate what they expect the addressees to do (Hood and Margetts 2007; John 2013; Lascoumes and Le Galès 2007). This is regularly the case when policymakers apply strategies for "NCD-prevention". But policymakers' considerations fail to address the situational parameters under which a person makes a decision; or in other words, and referring to Sunstein and Thaler (Thaler and Sunstein 2009), the design of the choice architecture. Considerations of this nature, however, are relevant and indeed vital if we wish to enhance the effectiveness of the instrument, especially when it comes to individual behaviour.

Furthermore, all these instruments follow a neoclassical rationality paradigm, according to which the complying actor (command-and-control instrument) calculates the prohibition and sanctions, and in which the calculating actor (incentive instrument) is probably the purest example of a rational actor, and in which the reasonable and intelligent actor (information/capacity instrument) acts after rationalising the individual or collective effects of non-compliance whereas the cooperative actor (organisation instrument) decides to collaborate with others when this is in his or her best interest. This paradigmatic view is especially evident in consumer policy and areas of that policy that have an impact on health (dietary habits, mobility behaviour, etc.). In these areas, policymakers often act on the assumption that the consumer is "sovereign" and only needs sufficient clear and detailed information to make decisions that are in his or her best interest. However, Reisch and Zhao show how this traditional view of policymaking contradicts the findings of behavioural sciences (Reisch and Zhao 2017, 192). It is important to understand that behavioural science does not proclaim the addressee to be "irrational" (as opposed to being rational) as such, but it shows that "heuristics and biases as well as situational dependency" play a role when it comes to decision-making (Reisch and Zhao 2017, 192).

Policy instruments are not always classified into the four groups mentioned; sometimes additional instruments are presented that extend this typology. In cases of government action that seeks to influence individual behaviour, Howlett (1991) suggests extending the typology by adding a category that he refers to as a "continuum model of instrument choice". This type of instrument defines "self-regulation" as an instrument that targets "private behaviour" (Howlett 1991, 12), which is typical of contemporary public health strategies at all policy levels. Since this is also the aim of regulatory, incentivising and capacity-building instruments, one might ask whether it actually represents a specific additional category of instruments. Following the argument set out in the paragraphs above, this chapter would suggest that self-regulation is an inherent part of the instruments presented. Interestingly enough, this view shows that Howlett in 1991 had already considered the fact that self-regulation is or may become the focus of policymaking and it leads us to the current debate on behavioural insights, which has become so important in public health. However, the aim of reinforcing "self-regulation" is also crucial when deciding on combining instruments or searching for new features that could reinforce established instruments. In accordance with Howlett's ideas on self-regulation (Howlett 1991) and his later remark on instruments that "directly affect the nature, types, quantities and distribution of the goods and services provided in society" (Howlett 2000, 415), it is useful to see the potential difference between instruments that focus on the individual, on the one hand, and, on the other hand, those that try to steer (corporate) organisations, like companies and interest groups—an aspect that Weaver also points out when he distinguishes between people as individuals, people as groups and other actors such as companies (Weaver 2016). But self-regulation and the focus on instruments are not the only aspects discussed in the literature.

In 2007—one year before Thaler and Sunstein published "Nudging" and the debate on their concept and behaviourally inspired policymaking began—Hood and Margetts wrote a remarkable passage in their book "The Tools of Government in the Digital Age":

> *Further […] the schema offered here draws attention to some instruments that are not easily classified under the headings of 'carrots, sticks and sermons' […] One notable example of a type of instrument that does not fit very readily into the 'carrots, sticks and sermons' (CSS) typology is the case where environments are physically structured so as to shape behaviour, […] fencing to shape crowd behaviour, for instance at sporting events or near pedestrian crossings on the road. This set of activities – sometimes called 'architecture' […] cannot really be forced into the 'CSS' trichotomy.* (C. C. Hood and Margetts 2007, 176).

Interestingly, they refer to Bentham and Foucault (governmentality) and explain that governments have been searching for such tools beyond "CSS". The technology of the digital age could help to construct such environments and (choice) architectures. Later, Hood and Margetts pointed out that the "the digital age may dramatically change the costs and practicality of different modes of action". The book ends with the diagnosis that "at the time of writing, the digital age is still at a relatively early stage" (C. C. Hood and Margetts 2007, 202). However, they were already spelling out the potential of digital techniques for governments in collecting and distributing information. This is the basis for governmental activities that observe how people behave, run trials ("randomised controlled trials", RCTs) and deduce policy inputs from the systematic analysis of human behaviour (test, learn, adapt, share)—activities that, for example, UK's Behavioural Insights Team (BIT) regularly applies. Such activities shall provide a basis for "evidence-based public health policy", which is already being discussed as a (future) trend (Brownson et al. 2009; Erwin and Brownson 2017), but at the same time accompanied by a critical debate on the nature and limits of such "evidence-based policy". Many people are participating in such observations voluntarily (e.g. wearables, health tracker). Although they are not (yet) part of governmental strategies, they are laying the groundwork for systematic data collection.

The systematic analysis of behaviour is linked to psychology and is in line with John, who puts psychology and communication at the centre of his contribution to the debate. John argues that "all tools are informational now" (see title of the article and John 2013, 616) and emphasises that "given the entrenched nature of the behaviours that governments wish to alter, such as eating habits, the driving of cars and energy use, the use of default and information cues on their own may not be enough to shift behaviour and outcomes" (John 2013, 612). John classifies "nudging" as a complement to conventional policy instruments and emphasises the blurring of the line between these instruments. Finally, he points out that how a policy affects the delivery is a question of communication and he refers to the "full range of psychological techniques" to achieve better results in policymaking (John 2013, 616). Furthermore, the aspect of "communication" is the focal point of his argument, as he concludes: "it makes more sense to regard tools as closely allied in the way they communicate preferred forms of behaviour" (John 2013, 616). We agree with the argument that behaviourally inspired instruments, especially nudging, are based mainly on information. Governments are therefore observing and experimenting to find new ways of nudging or influencing people's behaviour. The government's role as "detector" (C. C. Hood and Margetts 2007) is becoming ever more important, but in the context of this book we would argue that detecting the addressee's behaviour is key. Behavioural insights add a new spin in public policy (described as "enzymatic effect", see Loer 2018), which enables policymakers to boost the effectiveness of policy instruments.

In this way, the discussion on the use of behavioural insights in policymaking changes the view of the addressee since it deals directly with the question of how addressees behave and how behaviour and habits can be influenced. The use of nudging and behavioural insights in ways that suggest a new kind of intervention impacts on the traditional instruments themselves. Furthermore, this chapter argues that it brings a specific behavioural spin, rather than necessarily constituting a new, distinct and separate category of instruments. Such a new view of policymaking, which starts from a better understanding of people's behaviour, seems to be essential to tackling future challenges in public health policy. Some examples from public health show what can happen to instruments when they are infused with behavioural insights and given a behavioural spin.

Conclusions and (Future) Perspectives: Are Behavioural Insights the Key to Wicked Problems in Public Health?

Given the complexity of public health issues that preoccupy policymakers in many countries and international organisations (e.g. WHO, OECD), and considering the limits and coins of policy instruments, policymakers could either despair or search for innovative solutions and explore new avenues. Such new avenues would mean to give up linear causal thinking and top-down policymaking. Instead policymakers would acknowledge complexity science paradigms (Braithwaite et al. 2018). Following this perspective challenges not only the political science discourse on instruments, but even more political practice in public health: policy instruments and their combination—infused with behavioural insights or not—would have to be set up as "complexity-informed approaches" (Braithwaite et al. 2018, 8) and move away from idealistic pipeline models.

When it comes to NCDs and their complex causes and influencing factors, at least it seems as if the "classical" instruments—which follow such a pipeline model—have run into a wall since the major threats (e.g. obesity, heart conditions) persist or are even steadily increasing. Actually, causes (here: policies) and effects (here: rise or decline of epidemiologic figures) are not definitely connected and public health challenges part of a multidimensional system. It is impossible to evaluate how public health would have developed without the policies applied (e.g. education) or vice versa. Nevertheless, policymakers search for tools that would not provoke too much political opposition. In liberal democracies, not only do people want to decide on their own diet and lifestyles, they also want to be free to access substances that can lead to adverse health effects ("the dose makes the poison"). And in liberal democracies, companies want the right to defend their markets and revenues, and there are huge political obstacles to intervention in the market.

What solutions might there be for liberal democracies which—generally speaking—want to preserve freedom of choice? Behavioural science produces insights that could help policymakers to answer that question while acknowledging the conditions of liberal market societies—"nudging" might be one way to cope with the political challenges. "A subsidy is not a nudge; a tax is not a nudge; a fine or a jail sentence is not a nudge. To count as such, a nudge must preserve freedom of choice" (Sunstein 2017, 1). Starting from this definition, and studying the cases that Sunstein and others present (see Sunstein 2014 for a beautiful collection of examples), we can learn that "nudges" are related, at least, to "capacity" and "organisation". Capacity-building is part of a multitude of examples from the portfolio of "nudging", but it differs markedly from previous and familiar "capacity" (informational) approaches which have normally overlooked how people usually behave and which factors are involved in behaviour and decision-making. The US government, for example, introduced "myplate.gov" which helps people to diversify their daily diet in accordance with modern nutritional guidelines (Sunstein 2014, 76). This USDA Food Plate took the place of the "Food Pyramid", which was used for general informational guidance but caused misunderstandings and confusion (Sunstein 2014, 75). The differences between the two were the result of systematic, state-of-the-art research into human behaviour. Interestingly, it could be easily changed again if future research concludes that a different division of nutrition would be healthier. To sum up, behavioural sciences come up with insights that make people's decisions easier. A whole host of examples refer to disclosure requirements, which can be extremely effective, such as routinely informing parents of their child's BMI, accompanied by information about the relationship between BMI and health status. Referring to OIRA's work under the Obama administration, Sunstein also mentions "public-private partnerships" and the promotion of "international regulatory cooperation". "Public-private partnerships" are gaining attention when it comes to programmes like "Let's move", the "National School Lunch Program" or other initiatives implemented in schools and other public institutions. The companies that fit vending machines in schools have a direct impact on student's everyday eating habits since what they offer can tempt them into eating too much sugar and/or fat, or—if these machines are equipped with healthier products—could promote healthier alternatives. The setting of smart defaults is a further well-documented concept that has profited from behavioural science.

All in all, we would concur with Loewenstein and Chater, who see nudges as "a single concrete and powerful illustration of a much broader range of behaviourally-informed policy tools" (Loewenstein and Chater 2017, 28), but we would add that nudges cover a wide range of different tools, as seen in the examples above. To some extent, the debate on nudging and behavioural insights helps us to resolve the issue of the structural "blaming" of individuals for their shortcomings, since nudges are generally an attempt to create a choice architecture by which people can make better choices for themselves. This may be useful for public health if the design of instruments begins with the question of what is best for citizens if governments expect them to decide in a specific way.[6] It is possible to link well-established research that provides explanations for the emergence of specific health problems with the choice of instruments, and in doing so

[6] The expectation as such—or the political aim—has to be part of a different debate.

combine the structural and the individual dimension. This does not mean that the regulator should close its eyes to the "root cause of structural problems" (Loewenstein and Chater 2017, 33). Although the political obstacles might be significant, public health still needs to consider strict and coercive forms of regulation when tackling the social determinants of health. Since eating habits are a major issue in fighting NCDs, we would accept the argument of Loewenstein and Chater: "what we need, then, are regulations or taxes and subsidies that realign the food industry's incentives so that businesses internalise the health consequences that they are helping to propagate in terms of individuals and society (e.g. rising healthcare costs). Faced with incentives that are more closely aligned with their customers' interests, and with those of society as a whole, the food industry may decide to channel its considerable creativity into offering healthy and palatable products" (Loewenstein and Chater 2017, 37). In several publications, Sunstein shows how we can achieve the goal of channelling the food industry's activities in a healthier direction and how to initiate forms of intelligent cooperation (cp. various campaigns in the US, and the activities of the BIT, e.g. "LazyTown").

However, there are, of course, limits and coins associated with behaviourally informed instruments in public health, and it is fairly easy to identify advantages and disadvantages for every instrument or instrument mix. Voluntary agreements or commitments, for example, have their limits (for the example of reducing trans fatty acids see Knai et al. 2017) and require specific conditions to be effective. But when combined with "classical" instruments, they offer a chance to change both the social environment and the individual behaviour that occurs in that environment, by focusing on building a choice architecture that promotes healthier behaviours.

References

Asch, S. M., Stoto, M., Mendes, M., Valdez, R. B., Gallagher, M. E., Halverson, P., et al. (2005). A review of instruments assessing public health preparedness. *Public Health Reports, 120*(5), 532–542.

Böcher, M. (2012). A theoretical framework for explaining the choice of instruments in environmental policy. *Forest Policy and Economics, 16*, 14–22.

Böcher, M., & Töller, A. E. (2016). Inherent dynamics and chance as drivers in environmental policy? An approach to explaining environmental policy decisions. *submitted to Environmental Politics*, 1–27.

Braithwaite, J., Churruca, K., Long, J. C., Ellis, L. A., & Herkes, J. (2018). When complexity science meets implementation science: A theoretical and empirical analysis of systems change. *BMC Medicine, 16*(63), 1–14.

Brownell, K. D., & Warner, K. E. (2009). The perils of ignoring history: Big Tobacco played dirty and millions died. How similar is big food? *The Milbank Quarterly, 87*(1), 259–294. https://doi.org/10.1111/j.1468-0009.2009.00555.x.

Brownson, R. C., Chriqui, J. F., & Stamatakis, K. A. (2009). Understanding evidence-based public health policy. *American Journal of Public Health, 99*(9), 1576–1583.

Erwin, P. C., & Brownson, R. C. (2017). Macro trends and the future of public health practice. *Annual Review of Public Health, 38*, 393–412.

Evans, R. G., Barer, M. L., & Marmor, T. R. (1994). *Why are some people healthy and others not? The determinants of the health of populations*. Berlin/New York: Walter de Gruyter.

Hood, C. C. (1983). *The tools of government*. London: Palgrave Macmillan.

Hood, C. C., & Margetts, H. Z. (2007). *The tools of government in the digital age*. Basingstoke: Palgrave Macmillan.

Howlett, M. (1991). Policy instruments, policy styles, and policy implementation. *Policy Studies Journal, 19*(2), 1–21.

Howlett, M. (2000). Managing the "hollow state": Procedural policy instruments and modern governance. *Canadian Public Administration, 43*(4), 412–431.

Howlett, M. (2016). Policy tools & their targets: Beyond nudges and utility maximization in policy compliance. *IPSA, 2016*, 1–30.

Jann, W., & Wegrich, K. (2007). Theories of the policy cycle. In F. Fischer, G. J. Miller, & M. S. Sidney (Eds.), *Handbook of public policy analysis: Theory, politics, and methods* (pp. 43–62). Boca Raton: Taylor & Francis.

John, P. (2013). All tools are informational now: How information and persuasion define the tools of government. *Policy & Politics, 41*(4), 605–620.

Jordan, A., Wurzel, R. K., & Zito, A. (2005). The rise of 'new' policy instruments in comparative perspective: Has governance eclipsed government? *Political studies, 53*(3), 477–496.

Kickbusch, I. (2007). Responding to the health society. *Health Promotion International, 22*(2), 89–91.

Kingdon, J. W. (1995). *Agenda's, alternatives, and public policies*. Michigan: Harper Collins College Publishers.

Kirschen, E.-S. (1969). *Financial integration in Western Europe*. New York: Columbia University Press.

Knai, C., James, L., Petticrew, M., Eastmure, E., Durand, M., & Mays, N. (2017). An evaluation of a public–private partnership to reduce artificial trans fatty acids in England, 2011–16. *The European Journal of Public Health, 27*(4), 605–608.

Knill, C., & Lenschow, A. (2005). Compliance, competition and communication: Different approaches of European governance and their impact on national institutions. *JCMS: Journal of Common Market Studies, 43*(3), 583–606.

Lascoumes, P., & Le Galès, P. (2007). Introduction: Understanding public policy through its instruments – From the nature of instruments to the sociology of public policy instrumentation. *Governance, 20*(1), 1–21.

de Leeuw, E. (2017). Engagement of sectors other than health in integrated health governance, policy, and action. *Annual Review of Public Health, 28*, 329–349.

de Leeuw, E., Hoeijmakers, M., & Peters, D. T. (2016). Juggling multiple networks in multiple streams. *European Policy Analysis, 2*, 196–217. https://doi.org/10.18278/epa.2.1.13.

Lehner, M., Mont, O., & Heiskanen, E. (2015). Nudging: A promising tool for sustainable consumption behaviour? *Journal of Cleaner Production, 134*(Part A), 166–177. https://doi.org/10.1016/j.jclepro.2015.11.086.

Loer, K. (2018). The enzymatic effect of behavioural sciences – What about policymaker's expectations? In S. Beck & H. Strassheim (Eds.), *Handbook on behavioural change and public policy*. Cheltenham: Edward Elgar. Online: https://papers.ssrn.com/sol3/papers.cfm?abstract_id=3193655

Loewenstein, G., & Chater, N. (2017). Putting nudges in perspective. *Behavioural Public Policy, 1*(1), 26–53.

Lowi, T. (1972). Four systems of policy, politics, and choice. *Public Administration Review, 32*(4), 298–310.

Milio, N. (1981). *Promoting health through public policy*. Philadelphia: F. A. Davis Company.

Nathanson, C. A. (1999). Social movements as catalysts for policy change: The case of smoking and guns. *Journal of Health Politics, Policy & Law, 24*(3), 421–488.

Purnell, J. Q., Simon, S., Zimmermann, E. B., Camberos, G. J., & Fields, R. (2016). Policy implications of social determinants of health. In A. A. Eyler, J. F. Chriqui, S. Moreland-Russel, & R. C. Brownson (Eds.), *Prevention, policy, and public health* (pp. 93–114). New York: Oxford University Press.

Reisch, L. A., & Zhao, M. (2017). Behavioural economics, consumer behaviour and consumer policy: State of the art. *Behavioural Public Policy, 1*(2), 190–206.

Richardson, B. (2015). *Sugar*. Cambridge/Malden: Polity Press.

Rosen, G. (2015). *A history of public health*. Baltimore: Johns Hopkins University Press.

Schneider, A., & Ingram, H. (1990). Behavioral assumptions of policy tools. *The Journal of Politics, 52*(02), 510–529.

Sunstein, C. R. (2014). *Simpler: The future of government*. New York: Simon and Schuster.

Sunstein, C. R. (2017). *Misconceptions about nudges. Available at SSRN:* https://ssrn.com/abstract=3033101 *or* https://doi.org/10.2139/ssrn.3033101

Thaler, R. H., & Sunstein, C. R. (2008). *Nudge: Improving decisions about health, wealth, and happiness*. New Haven: Yale University Press.
Thaler, R. H., & Sunstein, C. R. (2009). *Nudge. Improving decisions about health, wealth, and happiness*. New York: Penguin.
Töller, A. E. (2013). The rise and fall of voluntary agreements in German environmental policy. *German Policy Studies, 9*(2), 49.
Töller, A. E. (2017). Voluntary regulation by the pharmaceutical industry – Which role for the shadow of hierarchy and social pressure? *European Policy Analysis, 3*(1), 48–80.
Vedung, E. (2003). Policy instruments: Typologies and theories. In M.-L. Bemelmans-Videc, R. C. Rist, & E. Vedung (Eds.), *Carrots, sticks & sermons. Policy instruments and their evaluation*. (pp. 21–58). New Brunswick/ New Jersey: Transaction Publishers. http://www.gbv.de/dms/bowker/toc/9780765805461.pdf.
Verweij, M. F., & Houweling, H. (2014). What is the responsibility of national government with respect to vaccination? *Vaccine, 32*(52), 7163–7166.
Weaver, R. K. (2016). *Encouraging longer working lives: A behavioural perspective*. Paper for ECPR Joint Sessions, Pisa 2016. Georgetown University and the Brookings Institution.

CHAPTER 4

Healthy Nations: Behavioural Approaches in Public Health Policy

Jessica Pykett

Abstract This chapter explores the rise of behavioural approaches to public health policies in different nation-states, exploring these in the context of contrasting efforts to address the social and spatial determinants of health and well-being. It examines how moral and political arguments for health promotion have given way to 'simpler' health strategies, albeit those which are based on increasingly sophisticated evidence and data relating to human behaviour and decision-making. In highlighting place-based and geographically variable understandings of health inequalities, the chapter considers how behavioural public health policies, which are growing in global significance, recast notions of health citizenship and governance towards behavioural, universal and marketised ideals. Using case studies from Singapore, the UK and the USA, the chapter explores the wider ethics of the behavioural turn in terms of its unintended consequences, its long-term sustainability and its capacity to transform health inequalities in different geographical contexts.

Keywords Public policy • Urban health • Social determinants of health • Lifestyles • Practices • Human geography

J. Pykett (✉)
University of Birmingham, Birmingham, UK
e-mail: J.Pykett@bham.ac.uk

B. Ewert, K. Loer (eds.), *Behavioural Policies for Health Promotion and Disease Prevention*, Palgrave Studies in Public Health Policy Research, https://doi.org/10.1007/978-3-319-98316-5_4

Introduction: Behavioural Approaches in Public Health Policy

> Although the conditions in which people are born, live and work are very important for their health, around half of the global burden of disease arises from behavioural and lifestyle factors. (Hallsworth et al. 2016)

The application of behavioural science research findings in public health governance has a long history which can sometimes be overlooked in the rush to declare as novel the solutions proposed by behavioural insights approaches to public health. Since the 1980s, the World Health Organisation has promoted behavioural change interventions including social marketing techniques. These techniques set out to address disease prevention and transmission, nutrition, hygiene and birth control, in response to calls from healthcare workers to address these seemingly intractable problems (WHO 1993a). In 1993, the WHO published learning modules for medical students on behavioural science evidence, with a focus on the 'prevention of disease by reducing unhealthy behaviours, improving treatment by changing a patient's behaviour, community diagnosis to identify high risk groups and areas, as well as behaviour change in health workers for greater effectiveness' (WHO 1993b, 2). It is no coincidence that the pioneers of the application of behavioural insights in public health have been in the global development sector, given the valued status of anthropological expertise within international NGOs. So too, these approaches fit historically with the socially paternalistic, and yet often economically liberalising frames of international development initiatives in general, which are found by some to be infantilising (Berndt and Boeckler 2017). Until recently, the focus of health policy in the Global South has been on communicable diseases such as Malaria, HIV/AIDS and TB. But since the early 2000s, there has been a worldwide emphasis on tackling non-communicable diseases (NCDs) (cancer, cardiovascular disease, diabetes and chronic respiratory disease) and their associated risk factors (tobacco, diet, physical activity, alcohol) (Herrick 2014, provides an overview of recent global public health policy trajectories).[1]

[1] The exception here is Tobacco use and its role in causing cancer, which was identified in the 1950s and put on the global health agenda in 1964 (see Herrick 2014, 186; Porter 1999, 299).

The rise of behavioural-insight-based approaches to public health, as justified in this chapter's opening quotation from a UK Behavioural Insights Team report, could thus be considered as a continuation of a gradual shift towards 'lifestyle' factors in public health policy. This is part of a long-term move towards health promotion and addressing the behaviour of the citizen as a matter of consumer choice. Indeed, it has been well established by historians of public health (Porter 1999; Rosen 2015 [1958]) that post-industrial nations in particular have witnessed a wholesale shift away from social policies aimed at reducing the effects of structural deprivation, for instance 19th-century public hygiene and sanitation infrastructures: tackling air pollution; providing clean water; sewerage and refuse collection. In the UK, the post-war establishment of the National Health Service, sickness benefits and the welfare state continued the state's strong role in the provision of conditions for basic health. These provisions have been replaced by what historian, Dorothy Porter (1999, 298) has described polemically as '[p]ropaganda campaigning now aimed to influence social behaviour and to educate citizens into adopting healthy lifestyles'. Post-industrial public health policies reveal a particular vision of healthful citizenship and demonstrate a specific social contract between citizen and state, shifting the locus of responsibility squarely onto the individual.

Notwithstanding these continuities, three features of current behavioural insights for public health policies indicate a shift in emphasis. The first is that moral and political arguments for the promotion of healthy lifestyles have given way to behavioural evidence which is used to justify an avowedly 'simple' public health strategy. Secondly, these behavioural explanations are said to be universal human qualities (deficiencies in cognition, behavioural biases) and are thus placed somewhat beyond the scope of political argumentation or geographical variability. Thirdly, where behavioural insights are prioritised above place-based accounts of health and disease, the social and structural aspects of health inequality, not least the failure of marketised public health agendas to address health inequalities, are side-lined. This chapter explores the significance of these shifts for understanding the relationship between health and governance, using case studies from three countries. It considers how behavioural, universal and market-driven solutions are dependent on an intentionally simplistic and naïve account of the politics of public health, a narrowing of the contextual or spatial drivers of health inequalities and a blinkered view of the types of evidence and disciplinary resources which could be marshalled to provide a more realistic diagnosis of ill-health and health inequalities and to shape more effective and sustainable public health policies in the future.

Healthful Nations, Healthful Citizens: Geographical Variation in Behavioural Public Health Policies

Some of the public health initiatives which have been informed by behavioural science and/or tested using behavioural science methods such as randomised controlled trials (RCTs) are highly morally or politically controversial in their specific national contexts. One example is the use of default 'opt-out' procedures for organ donation, which is soon to be implemented in the UK after long delays and despite opposition, and which several other countries worldwide have already put in place. A second example is the failed proposal of former New York Mayor, Michael Bloomberg, to restrict the sale of super-sized soda drinks (he was later successful in introducing a sugar tax in Cook County, Illinois—which became the subject of a political battle and multi-million-dollar advertising campaign (Jaspen 2017)). Despite clear evidence that these behaviourally informed public policies save lives and do not ultimately restrict individual freedom (people can still choose to withdraw consent, or buy several 'regular' sized sugary drinks), these examples have sometimes fallen short of the level of public acceptability that would be required for their introduction in specific countries. However, the majority of health initiatives supported by behavioural insights units around the world are in fact relatively benign: the placement of fruit at eye level in supermarkets; the increased prominence of healthy meal options in schools; the use of social norm prompts in reducing missed hospital appointments. There is a rapidly expanding repertoire of contemporary behavioural techniques used for health promotion, many examples of which are pragmatic, sensible and measured options for public health policy (see Chap. 3).

It is only when we take a longer-term perspective on these techniques that we can begin to consider their political and historical significance. These apparently small, detailed and context-specific initiatives can be said to have a significant cumulative effect. David Halpern, Chief Executive of the UK's Behavioural Insights Team refers to this as a 'radical incrementalism' (2015, 291), of which he argues: '…we can be pretty confident that each of these incremental improvements can lead to an overall performance that is transformative in its cost-effectiveness and impact'. This chapter focuses on the connection between these politically neutral narratives of cost-effectiveness, an evidential base, real-world relevance and simplicity, and the cumulative impact of behaviourally informed public health policies on the practices of health governance and healthful citizenship. It examines the way in which policymakers in different countries are drawing on these narratives to address complex health problems, and outlines some of the public controversies that have followed. The chapter thus explores the political claims-making and broader ethical effects that are indicated by behavioural forms of health governance. In so doing, we can begin to think afresh about whether place and practice-based approaches are a fitting response to the urgent public health challenges that we collectively face.

Doing 'What Works' in the UK: Charges of the Nannystate

The UK is often considered as the front-runner in terms of developing behavioural approaches to public policy in general, and behavioural health policies in particular. Since the early 2000s, there has been an open debate about the potential benefit of 'behaviour change' approaches to policy, with influential policy strategists advising a shift towards personal responsibility (Halpern et al. 2004). During this time, within public health, social marketing experts were employed by the National Health Service (NHS), and 'NHS Choices' (the public-facing health information website of the NHS) incorporated many behavioural insights, such as targeting segmented audiences in its anti-obesity communications strategies, highlighting social norms to reduce alcohol use, and designing interventions which took advantage of key life stages, timeframes and pre-stated commitments to promote new healthy habits or lifestyle changes such as quitting smoking (DoH 2011). By 2010, the Behavioural Insights Team (BIT) had been set up within the Cabinet Office, in order to promote and coordinate behavioural science approaches across government departments and to trial policy initiatives and interventions which experimented with administrative procedures, communications techniques and existing regulations in order to change policy outcomes. In short, the BIT used what behavioural economists and psychologists knew about the biases, frames and cues for human behaviour, rejecting the rationality assumption of traditional economic thinking, to make public policy more effective, and—crucially at a time of government spending cuts—less costly (see Jones et al. 2013;

Halpern 2015 for accounts of the institutional history of the BIT and behavioural economics).

With the increasing momentum that was derived from positive evidence gained through many of the BIT's trials, and the growing influence of the BIT and behavioural forms of governance around the world (Lourenço et al. 2016; OECD 2017a; Whitehead et al. 2014; World Bank 2015), the UK's public health sector has embraced nudges, tactical interventions and experimental trials, as evidenced by the commitment of the UK's second largest public health charity, the Health Foundation to fund a Behavioural Insights Research Programme of over £3 million since 2015. In government too, in the context of what most see as the chronic underfunding of the NHS, the Conservative government's NHS Five Year Forward Review (2014) advances a particularly experimental approach, for instance, by investing in new health technologies, supporting '"test bed" sites for world innovators', 'new "green field" sites where completely new NHS services will be designed from scratch' (NHS 2014, 5), and work on 'behavioural "nudge" type policies in health care' (NHS 2014, 35). In the absence of significant clinical evidence on the efficacy of nudges in healthcare (Marteau et al. 2011; McDaid and Merkur 2014), the latter may seem a risky strategy. One might also question just how novel and experimental the Five Year Forward Review is, given commitments long associated with Conservative governments in the UK to open up the NHS to global healthcare companies ('world innovators'), and to apportion responsibility for ill-health to individuals themselves in a manner which has long been criticised by legal scholars and bioethicists (Brown 2013; Crawshaw 2013). As the Review clearly sets out:

> we live longer, with complex health issues, sometimes of our own making. One in five adults still smoke. A third of us drink too much alcohol. Just under two thirds of us are overweight or obese. (NHS 2014, 2)

This emphasis on prevention and personal responsibility has been a well-established feature of successive UK government's approaches to public health since at least the 1970s (Kelly and Russo 2017, 3), so it is difficult to discern anything of a step-change here. What is most significant about the most recent calls for the application of behavioural insights to health may instead be the way in which they propose new sources of evidence for justifying behavioural solutions, while rehearsing older narratives about the 'lifestyle' drivers of ill-health. Thus a set of intractable political-economic problems which affect deeply and systematically the provision of healthcare and the persistence of health inequalities are re-framed in terms of the behaviour of individuals. It has been argued that this 'simple narrative' is attractive to policy makers who seek short-term simple solutions without confronting the vested interests of the industries involved in producing risky conditions for health, and that such a narrative is dependent on a fundamentally mistaken conflation of disease causation and prevention, and an absence of policy designed to address the social determinants of health (Kelly and Russo 2017, 3). In the UK, at least, the consequence of these narratives is often that public and political debate focuses on critiquing a perceived loss of autonomy; bemoaning the 'nanny' state (Jochelson 2006; Lansley 2010) which is telling us to stop drinking, smoking and eating tasty foods. This consideration of autonomy is not, however, sufficient in assessing the ethics of behavioural insights in public health (Blumenthal-Barby and Burroughs 2012; Verweij and van den Hoven 2012; Oliver 2015).

If we are to consider the ethics of *responsibility* rather than autonomy, we get a more accurate account of issues of substantive freedoms, capability and culpability. As such, we can consider lifestyle factors alongside the underfunding of public health services and other sources of contemporary ill-health. These might include over-consumption encouraged by a deregulated and highly industrialised food and drink industry, the over-availability and advertising of health-harming products (Rayner and Lang 2011) and overworking, including long hours and workplace stress (Carter et al. 2013; Sparks et al. 1997). That these kinds of structural, contextual and demographically uneven issues are rarely tackled by behaviourally informed health policies has led public health critics to argue that 'nudge becomes collusion between the state and corporations to hoodwink consumers' (Rayner and Lang 2011, 899). The voluntary 'responsibility deals' struck between government and the food and drink industry in the UK are an infamous example of weak and ineffective policy in this area. In this sense, even if behavioural public health policies draw on the best available evidence about what works in health promotion and prevention (though even this is strongly disputed) (Baum and Fisher 2014; Kelly and Russo 2017), wider democratic and moral arguments about the locus of responsibility for public health remain outside of the parameters of discussion.

Changing Singaporean Habits: Lifestyle Approaches in Context

Singapore—as city-state often noted for its innovation—was quick to adopt behavioural insights in public policy. Institutions such as the Civil Service College (CSC), Singapore Management University, the Lee Kuan Yew School of Public Policy (LKY), the Design Thinking Unit and The Human Experience Lab in the Prime Minister's Public Service Division, Behavioural Insights units within various government ministries and a cadre of social enterprises and policy-focused start-ups have been exploring the value of behavioural approaches since 2011. The UK's BIT provided direct advice to government agencies, and launched its own branch office in Singapore in 2016. The head of the Singaporean Civil Service, Peter Ong praised nudge approaches at the global 'Behavioural Exchange' conference held in Singapore, 2017. All this signifies a concerted effort and a high-level enthusiasm to explore the potential for integrating behavioural insights into government policy, although there is currently no central office at the executive level whose primary purpose has been to coordinate a behavioural approach.

Within Singapore's health sector, there have been default opt-out settings for health insurance plans (Medishield) since the 1980s, and there is opt-out for organ donation, following public consultation. This suggests that Singapore was an early adopter of behavioural insights in healthcare, although these measures were not necessarily informed by behavioural economics. Indeed, in this one-party state, the government does not shy away from strong mandatory regulation, and in 2015 legislation was passed to make Medishield compulsory, with action taken against those who fail to sign up. In this sense, while enthusiastic about nudges, the Singaporean state is not necessarily committed to the *politically libertarian* paternalistic values which are said to underpin nudges. A more explicit example of behavioural insights in health is found in the work of the Health Promotion Board, which has played a key role in preventative, lifestyle-based health campaigns. One such example is the Million KG Challenge, a weight-loss initiative that supports participants in getting started with healthy eating and physical activity, using the principles of gamification to reward them with vouchers and prizes, and buddying up participants with friends to keep them motivated. As Peter Ong (2015) described it: 'the Million KG Challenge nudges each participant towards their weight-loss goal by making goals salient and achievable at each stage'. Similarly to the UK's emphasis on lifestyle health factors, lack of willpower is identified as one of the key drivers of the unwarranted financial burden on the health system. The Million KG Challenge is one of several initiatives undertaken by the Health Promotion Board which recognise the inadequacy of information to ensure behavioural changes. Rather, the emphasis is now on 'influencing', taking account of 'behavioural traits such as how Singaporeans think, decide and form new habits' (Tan et al. 2017).

In Singapore, as elsewhere, this includes attention to the environmental cues which shape healthy and unhealthy decisions, such as the availability of unhealthy options when dining out. The Healthier Dining Programme, for instance, worked with food and beverage providers, mapping where Singaporeans were most likely to eat out, and working in partnership with these companies to market healthier choices, promotions and point-of-sale prompts (Tan et al. 2017, 47). As such, the external context is said to be as important as the inner workings of the mind in shaping everyday decisions, a prevalent notion in behavioural approaches to health (Hollands et al. 2016). This may include the size of portions or serving plates, the way that information is displayed, the design of canteens and cafes, the attractiveness of taking the stairs instead of the lift; in short, the 'choice architectures' which are already infused in the contexts in which we think, decide and act. However, when we start to expand our definition of 'context' away from the immediate perceptual environment and towards the political, economic, social and cultural context in which nudges are offered as health policy solutions in the first place, it is possible to take a more geographically specific view of the significance of behavioural insights in health. In doing so, we can begin to generate new questions about the ethics and politics of health nudges, not in simple terms of interference—or otherwise—by a nannying state, but in terms of the potential effects on the ground of cumulative interventions in the lives and environs of citizens.

Ironically, it is within the 'flawed democracy' of Singapore (The Economist 2016 Democracy Index[2]), famed for its sometimes authoritarian state interference in the 'graciousness', littering and personal behaviour of its citizens, that some of the limitations and dangers of health nudges are increasingly the focus of public debate. It might be considered somewhat incongruent that the Singapore Government has embraced potentially liberalising nudges conceived in the context of the USA, where

[2] https://www.eiu.com/public/topical_report.aspx?campaignid=DemocracyIndex2016

citizens are inherently suspicious of 'big government', and trialled in the UK, during an unprecedented period of state retrenchment—issues which are largely anathema to a Singaporean context. Policy strategists, academics and young policy entrepreneurs alike have commented on this irony, noting for instance that the high levels of trust placed in government agencies to operate efficiently, the stereotyped social compliance of Singaporean citizens, the size and manageability of the city-state and the lack of political alternatives, might all suggest that nudges and RCTs might not be necessary; the Singapore state will effectively do what it wants (Whitehead et al. 2017, 102). All the more surprising, therefore, that Singaporean social scientists have begun to question whether all these small nudges in health policy and elsewhere are really good for society. In a recent article in the magazine of Singapore's CSC, Walter Theseira and Ong Qiyan (2017) consider the 'hidden costs' of nudging, highlighting the need to weigh up the welfare benefits of nudging with the unintended costs of potentially leading 'people to make choices that are inconsistent with their own preferences or interests'. This may include universal approaches to health promotion which may inadvertently cause harm or emotionally impact those who are not at fault:

> negative messaging is increasingly being considered to address other health-related issues, such as sedentary lifestyles, obesity, and the consumption of sugar, meat, and fat. Those who have no serious health problems will likely resent being made to feel guilty or shameful at the occasional indulgence. Others, who are trying hard to improve their habits, may likewise feel shame and stigma. (Theseira and Qiyan 2017, 71)

Indeed, their broader point is that the 'radical incrementalism' of small nudges described by Halpern above can indeed have transformative impacts, and that these have not been considered or understood to the same evidential standards as those prescribed by the behavioural science on which they are based. They caution that:

> Every behavioural intervention that is narrowly focused on a specific policy goal may impose a small, but cumulative, cognitive tax on members of the public. A barrage of such nudges may gradually deplete our capacity to plan and make good decisions. (Theseira and Qiyan 2017, 73)

As others have already argued (Jones et al. 2010; Jones et al. 2013; Hausman and Welsh 2010), the fundamental basis of behavioural insights for health is the inadequacy of informational/educational approaches to change behaviour. This inadequacy is related to a plethora of psychological biases inherent to human decision-making and the pervasive influence of human ecologies which promote unhealthy living. Yet bypassing people's irrationalities, susceptibilities to influence and the drowning out of health lifestyle information in a world full of harmful corporate nudges may not empower citizens to act in healthier ways in the future. Therefore, an ethical approach to behavioural public health must necessarily consider more deeply the effects of health nudges on the empowerment, education and capabilities of individuals and societies to make better future decisions (Tengland 2012). In this context, we must take a closer look at the dominant framings and drivers of public (ill) health and decide whether we are asking the right questions and developing the most effective solutions.

Nudging America: A Failure to Address Market Failure

Part of the reason for the global success of behavioural public policy, according to Richard Thaler, co-author of *Nudge* (Thaler and Sunstein 2008), was the coincidence that Barak Obama was elected as President of the United States in 2008, later appointing his former colleague, and *Nudge's* co-author Cass Sunstein, as head of the White House Office of Information and Regulatory Affairs (Thaler 2015). In this position, Sunstein (2011) encouraged government agencies to incorporate behavioural insights into their policies, and a Social and Behavioural Sciences Team (SBST) was established in 2014—re-instating a sub-committee of the White House National Science and Technology Council originally chartered in 2004 (White House 2015). A year on, an executive order on 'Using Behavioral Science Insights to Better Serve the American People' was passed by the Obama administration. This order, among other things, was to enable 'Americans to lead longer, healthier lives', by simplifying administrative processes, improving the presentation of information for public programmes, including how choices could be arranged or defaulted to support and enhance welfare, and generally make desirable citizen action easier while also reducing regulatory burdens.[3]

[3] https://obamawhitehouse.archives.gov/the-press-office/2015/09/15/executive-order-using-behavioral-science-insights-better-serve-american

While it is not yet clear how widespread the policy ramifications of this order have been, there have been a number of health intervention research trials in the USA in which nudges have been evident. The New York Times, for instance, recently reported on trials in Pennsylvania for smoking cessation and weight-loss programmes which have used the behavioural economic principle of loss aversion to shape interventions involving people pledging their own money and getting it back only if they complete the programme (Khullar 2017). So too, new companies which combine behavioural insights with self-tracking health and fitness technologies have emerged to capitalise on the way in which healthful behaviour has become a lifestyle issue. One such company, NudgeCoach, has a mobile app which enables users to 'take back control of your health'.[4] Other companies such as those involved in the 'Blue Zones Project' have invited comparisons between nudges and place-based health promotion programmes. The Blue Zones Project began in Iowa in 2011, and is a community and place-based public health promotion initiative based on the work of author, Dan Buettner (Carter 2015). Buettner travelled the globe in search of places where people lived longer, in order to identify the lifestyle and environmental conditions necessary for improving health. Online lifestyle quizzes and calculators, group seminars and events, advice on diet, relationships and personal fulfilment and working with city authorities to develop environmental nudges to 'deconvenience' people's lives (getting people walking, having healthier restaurant options) are all combined to inspire Iowans to 'improve their health and happiness' (Healthiest State Initiative 2014, cited in Carter 2015, 378). It is not just health responsibility that is emphasised in these examples, but a promise of self-empowerment. Yet while the Blue Zones Project may seem a welcome intervention to promote community and individual action for health, Carter argues that its discourse, practices and funding regimes (healthcare insurance providers and wellness companies) are suggestive of the neoliberalisation of health promotion and the narrowing of political discussion of the social and structural determinants of health inequalities, and is almost entirely silent on the organisation, funding and infrastructure of hospitals and medical care (Carter 2015, 378).

In contrast to this apparently de-politicised programme of healthy lifestyle nudges, the highly politically contested *Affordable Care Act* (ACA,

[4] https://nudgecoach.com/nudgeapp/

known as Obamacare), is evidence of the limitations of the public acceptability of behaviourally informed policies in a manner which is quite specific to the US context. This is a context which appears (from a European perspective at least) to involve a rather self-defeating cultural loyalty to the 'freedom' to reject healthcare, and thus—put crudely—to run the risk of being ill without recourse to treatment except at great individual cost. The ACA aimed to increase health insurance coverage across the US while also reducing premiums, in light of the ongoing lack of access to medical care experienced particularly among low-income and non-white population groups (Chen et al. 2016). The ACA is not a nudge itself, since it clearly mandates people to purchase (now more highly subsidised) health insurance, and mandates providers to accept all applications for such insurance. Yet it is behaviourally informed, in the sense that it has tried to support and guide consumer decisions using the principles of choice architecture. First, the new default compulsory nature of the Act recognises that people tend to discount the future when making financial decisions in the present. Secondly, since people must choose from a large number of options, the ACA developed categories of plans (Bronze, Silver, Gold) to cover different eventualities. It has already been demonstrated that the Act has increased health insurance cover and reduced racial inequalities in such cover (Chen et al. 2016), but behavioural economists have highlighted that consumers are still not making the most cost-effective choices for them (Bhargava et al. 2017). The evidence they provide is consistent, they note, with the tendency of insurance providers to over-complicate products in ways which increase profits and decrease consumer welfare (Bhargava et al. 2017, 10).

The ACA thus offers a rather contradictory example of behaviourally informed health policy (both involving mandates and supporting choice), but it also highlights a key difference between countries in which the private sector dominates healthcare financing and those which are based on public infrastructures. On the one hand, the ACA—while ending the freedom to choose to be *not* insured—still operates within a largely liberal health insurance market. The behavioural 'tweaks' which have been embedded within the Act, while welcomed by consumer rights advocates, have arguably not addressed the key issue, which is the failure of the market to increase competition, drive down prices, drive up quality and ensure the health and welfare of citizens. This is indicative of the prioritisation of individual consumer choice over the stated goal of 'Better Serving the American People'. It is in part a result of the effective lack of collectivised responsibility for health, and in part a misidentification of the root causes of ill-health, as epitomised in the following quote from Harvard Medical School doctor, Dhruv Khullar, writing in the *New York Times*:

> Health is fundamentally the product of myriad daily decisions made by doctors and patients, and by uncovering what truly motivates us, we may be able to nudge one another toward wiser decisions and healthier lives.

Health is, of course, related to what doctors and patients do and how they act, but these actions cannot be properly evaluated and addressed out of context (Kelly and Russo 2018; Cohn and Lynch 2017). It is thus worth questioning whether nudging can offer anything but a sticking plaster to issues of public health in the context of the enduring ideological battleground over healthcare markets and affordability in the USA.

While the Trump administration may prove the death knell for both the White House SBST[5] and Obamacare, what these examples provide is an indication of the importance of national context—in terms of politics, economics and culture—to the shaping of behavioural public health policies, their likely long-term effects and the level of public acceptance of such policies, which will vary between nations (see Reisch et al. 2017). By focusing on national rather than personal differences, we can begin to unpick some of the simplifying logics of behavioural health policies and their relative silence on the social determinants of health inequality. Indeed, although the opening quote to this chapter maintains that behavioural factors account for half of global disease, the World Health Organisation itself now highlights the inadequacy of behavioural change for addressing global ill-health. They emphatically call for policy interventions to act on the circumstances of daily life and the structural drivers of health outcomes (Commission on Social Determinants of Health 2008, 42). Yet for some there is a clear political rationale for emphasising the behavioural determinants of health as explained by Baum and Fisher (2014, 218):

> There is a strong inherent logic to behavioural change strategies. If the problem of smoking is seen as one of people choosing to smoke and obesity as one of people over-eating, then telling them not to do this seems to make sense. This is a powerful, simple logic for politicians and does not involve upsetting corporate donors to political parties [...] or require legislative change that will inevitably attract complaints about a nanny state.

[5] Since 2017: https://oes.gsa.gov

Conclusion: *Place* and *Practice* Approaches to Public Health Promotion

This chapter has explored the increasing focus on lifestyle and behavioural approaches in public health policy emerging globally, considering the antecedents of this shift, and the emerging differences in the application of behavioural insights in health in different countries. It has highlighted that there is a tendency, where 'nudge' or behavioural public policies are promoted, to downplay other significant drivers of public health and health inequalities, and thus to simplify health problems as deserving of individual, administrative, (proximate) environmental and behavioural solutions—even if proponents of nudge are careful to point out that such policies are just one strand among a suite of policy tools available to governments.

Meanwhile, supranational bodies, among others, have recently called for further research on the ethics and effects of behavioural public policies, for an exploration of the potential for more empowering forms of behavioural governance, for a more pluralistic set of methodologies for evaluating policy impact, and for discussion on the regulatory architectures required to check the power and function of behavioural public policies (Jones et al. 2013; Lourenço et al. 2016; OECD 2017b). Bioethics, social science, medical sociology and histories of the human and psychological sciences could be usefully drawn on to set out future research agendas to meet these challenges, and yet it is predominantly behavioural scientists who are called upon to set the parameters of such endeavours.

In concluding, I want to outline an alternative approach to analysing behavioural public health policies which addresses the geographical variation in the drivers and effects of such policies, and to consider the active role of *place* and *practices* in shaping public health. In her discussion of global public health policies, Claire Herrick (2014) notes the renewal of the field of urban public health and urban political ecology as positive moves towards a more sophisticated analysis of the governance of health and health disparities. Herrick's call for a revival of a place-based approach to public health seeks to provide insight into 'the mechanisms linking urbanisation processes, urban management, the provision of basic infrastructure and services, planning, healthcare services, informality, employment, education, consumption and health outcomes' (Herrick 2014, 187). She argues that there is an ethical imperative for the field of public health to develop appropriate ways to study how global health funding, structures of governance, intervention techniques and local experience are connected—reflecting the call from urban political ecologists to investigate how apparently natural biophysical properties such as health have been commodified (Herrick 2014, 187). One way in which this might be done is through the engagement of behavioural scientists with critical policy scholars who have analysed public health policy discursively or anthropologically. A complementary route is to involve epidemiologists and geographers who have modelled *neighbourhood effects* on public health—to show how place-based structural and demographic factors shape health decisions and outcomes, in relation to smoking for instance (e.g. Duncan et al. 1999), or life-expectancy (Thomas et al. 2010).

Another approach is to consider *practice-based* and sociological accounts of health, in order to specify the conceptual and methodological assumptions underpinning the behavioural approach. In their evaluation of a nudge-based public health RCT in Cambridgeshire, UK, medical sociologists, Cohn and Lynch (2017, 3) argue that habits and automatic behaviours have come to dominate health psychology at the expense of wider considerations of context-based practices. While this fits well with a government commitment to autonomy preserving nudges, in effect, what they have found in their empirical research is evidence that people themselves adopt a rather different conception of habits, based more on everyday mundane routines and the contextual opportunities afforded to them to change or sustain particular socially embedded practices (Cohn and Lynch 2017, 8; see also Thompson et al. 2007). The 'simple experimental logic' of the RCT, by which all variables except for the intervention must be kept stable, thus has the perverse effect of 'designing out' context, separating the internal and external drivers of practices, and treating the experimental body as a static entity (Cohn and Lynch 2017, 2). In other words, the behavioural findings used to justify behavioural public health policies can be guilty of producing the artefacts of their own research assumptions. The combined contribution of these medical sociologists and health geographers is to highlight how place and context are more than a back-drop to behaviour, more than a set of environmental cues. Rather they are constitutive of health practices. To ignore this dynamic relation between place and people's health is likely to foreclose the development of public health policies which are effective and sustainable over the long term. Simple narratives, simplified experimental logics and simple solutions are rarely adequate in tackling the complex, multi-causal pathways of NCDs and the dynamic and unequal lives of individuals and social groups in different national contexts. Relying on the power of the market, through the modification of choice architectures and behavioural prompts will not radically transform global health outcomes and inequalities. Evaluating the long-term effectiveness, ethics and impact on the empowerment of diverse citizens of behavioural health policies is therefore an urgent priority for public health researchers.

References

Baum, F., & Fisher, M. (2014). Why behavioural health promotion endures despite its failure to reduce health inequities. *Sociology of Health & Illness, 36*(2), 213–225.

Berndt, C., & Boeckler, M. (2017). Economic, experiments, evidence: Poor behaviour and the development of market subjects. In V. Higgins & W. Larner (Eds.), *Assembling neoliberalism. Expertise, practices, subjects* (pp. 283–302). New York: Palgrave Macmillan.

Bhargava, S., Loewenstein, G., & Benartzi, S. (2017). The costs of poor health (plan choices) and prescriptions for reform. *Behavioural Science & Policy, 3*(1), 1–12.

Blumenthal-Barby, J. S., & Burroughs, H. (2012). Seeking better health care outcomes: The ethics of using the "nudge". *The American Journal of Bioethics, 12*(2), 1–10.

Brown, R. C. H. (2013). Moral responsibility for (un)healthy behaviour. *Journal of Medical Ethics., 39*, 695–698.

Carter, B., Danford, A., Howcroft, D., Richardson, H., Smith, A., & Taylor, P. (2013). 'Stressed out of my box': Employee experience of lean working and occupational ill-health in clerical work in the UK public sector. *Work, Employment and Society, 27*(5), 747–767.

Carter, E. D. (2015). Making the Blue Zones: Neoliberalism and nudges in public health promotion. *Social Science & Medicine, 133*, 374–382.

Chen, J., Vargas-Bustaante, A., Mortensen, K., & Ortega, A. N. (2016). Racial and ethnic disparities in health care access and utilization under the Affordable Care Act. *Medical Care, 54*(2), 140–146.

Cohn, S., & Lynch, R. (2017). Falling into a routine: From habits to situated practices. *Sociology of Health and Illness, 39*(8), 1–14. https://doi.org/10.1111/1467-9566.12597.

Commission on the Social Determinants of Health. (2008). *Closing the gap in a generation: Health equity through action on the social determinants of health.* Final Report of the Commission on Social Determinants of Health. Geneva: World Health Organization.

Crawshaw, P. (2013). Public health policy and the behavioural turn: The case of social marketing. *Critical Social Policy, 33*(4), 616–637.
Department of Health. (2011). *Changing behaviour, improving outcomes. A new social marketing strategy for public health*. London: Department of Health.
Duncan, C., Jones, K., & Moon, G. (1999). Smoking and deprivation: Are there neighbourhood effects? *Social Science & Medicine, 48*(4), 497–505.
Hallsworth, M., Snijders, V., Burd, H., Prestt, J., Judah, G., Huf, S., & Halpern, D. (Behavioural Insights Team). (2016). *Applying behavioural insights. Simple ways to improve health outcomes*. Doha: World Innovation Summit for Health.
Halpern, D. (2015). *Inside the nudge unit. How small changes can make a big difference*. London: WH Allen.
Halpern, D., Bates, C., Mulgan, G., Aldridge, S., Beales, G., & Heathfield, A. (2004). *Personal responsibility and changing behaviour: The state of knowledge and its implications for public policy*. London: Cabinet Office.
Hausman, D. M., & Welch, B. (2010). Debate: To nudge or not to nudge. *The Journal of Political Philosophy, 18*(1), 123–136.
Herrick, H. (2014). (Global) health geography and the post-2015 development agenda. *The Geographical Journal, 180*(2), 185–190.
Hollands, G. J., Marteau, T. M., & Fletcher, P. C. (2016). Non-conscious processes in changing health-related behaviour: A conceptual analysis and framework. *Health Psychology Review, 10*(4), 381–394.
Jaspen, B. (2017, September 1). Billionaire Bloomberg spends millions to rescue Chicago-area soda Tax. *Forbes*. Available at: https://www.forbes.com/sites/brucejapsen/2017/09/01/billionaire-bloomberg-spends-millions-to-save-chicago-area-soda-tax/#265be4b31238. Accessed 05 Oct 2017.
Jochelson, K. (2006). Nanny or steward? The role of government in public health. *Public Health, 120*(12), 1149–1155.
Jones, R., Pykett, J., & Whitehead, M. (2010). Big society's little nudges: The changing politics of health care in an age of austerity. *Political Insight, 1*(3), 85–87.
Jones, R., Pykett, J., & Whitehead, M. (2013). *Changing behaviours. On the rise of the psychological state*. Cheltenham: Edward Elgar.
Kelly, M., & Russo, F. (2018). Causal narratives in public health: The difference between mechanisms of aetiology and mechanisms of prevention in non-communicable diseases. *Sociology of Health and Illness, 40*(1), 1–18. https://doi.org/10.1111/1467-9566.12621.
Khullar, D. (2017, April 13). How behavioral economics can produce better health care. *New York Times*. Available at: https://www.nytimes.com/2017/04/13/upshot/answer-to-better-health-care-behavioral-economics.html. Accessed 28 Nov 2017.
Lansley, A. (2010). *Secretary of State for Health's speech to the UK Faculty of Public Health Conference – 'A new approach to public health'*. Available at http://webarchive.nationalarchives.gov.uk/+/http://www.dh.gov.uk/en/MediaCentre/Speeches/DH_117280. Accessed 28 Nov 2017.

Lourenço, J. S., Ciriolo, E., Almeida, R. S., & Troussard, X. (2016). *Behavioural insights applied to policy: European report*. EUR 27726 EN. https://doi.org/10.2760/903938.

Marteau, T., Ogilvie, D., Roland, M., Suhrcke, M., and Kelly, M. P. (2011, January 29). Judging nudging: Can nudging improve population health? *BMJ, 342*, 263–365.

McDaid, D., & Merkur, S. (2014). To nudge, or not to nudge, that is the question. *Eurohealth, 20*(2), 3–5.

National Health Service. (2014). *Five year forward view*. NHS England, at: https://www.england.nhs.uk/five-year-forward-view/. Accessed 14 Sept 2018.

OECD. (2017a). *Behavioural insights and public policy. Lessons from around the world*. Paris: OECD. Available at: http://www.oecd.org/gov/regulatory-policy/behavioural-insights-and-public-policy-9789264270480-en.htm. Accessed 28 Nov 2017.

OECD. (2017b, May). *Behavioural insights in public policy: Key messages and summary from OECD international events*. Paris: OECD. www.oecd.org/gov/regulatory-policy/OECD-events-behavioural-insights-summary-may-2017.pdf. Accessed 28 Nov 2017.

Oliver, A. (2015). Nudging, shoving, and budging: Behavioural economic-informed policy. *Public Administration, 93*(3), 700–714.

Ong, P. (2015). *Speech by Mr Peter Ong, head of civil service Singapore at "Frontiers of behavioural economics: Choice and well-being in the Asia Pacific"*. https://www.cscollege.gov.sg/About%20Us/newsroom/2015/Pages/Speech-by-Mr-Peter-Ong,-Head-of-Civil-Service-Singapore-at-Frontiers-of-Behavioural-Economics.aspx. Accessed 02 Nov 2017.

Porter, D. (1999). *Health, civilization and the state. A history of public health from ancient to modern times*. London: Routledge.

Rayner, G., & Lang, T. (2011). Is nudge an effective public health strategy to tackle obesity? No. *BMJ, 342*, d2177.

Reisch, L. A., Sunstein, C. R., & Gwozdz, W. (2017). Beyond carrots and sticks: Europeans support health nudges. *Food Policy, 69*, 1–10.

Rosen, G. (2015 [1958]). *A history of public health* (Revised expanded ed.). Baltimore: Johns Hopkins University Press.

Sparks, K., Cooper, C., Fried, Y., & Shirom, A. (1997). The effects of hours of work on health: A meta-analytic review. *Journal of Occupational and Organizational Psychology, 70*, 391–408.

Sunstein, C. (2011). Empirically informed regulation. *University of Chicago Law Review, 78*(4), 1349–1429.

Tan, V., Utravathy, V., & Ling, C. (2017). Healthy living, everyday. In *Ethos* 17 (pp. 44–51). Singapore: Civil Service College.

Tengland, P.-A. (2012). Behavior change or empowerment: On the ethics of health-promotion strategies. *Public Health Ethics, 5*(2), 140–153.

Thaler, R. (2015). Foreword. In D. Halpern (Ed.), *Inside the nudge unit*. London: W H Allen.

Thaler, R., & Sunstein, C. R. (2008). *Nudge. Improving decisions about health, wealth and happiness*. London: Yale University Press.

Theseira, W., & Qiyan, O. (2017). The hidden costs of behavioural interventions. In *Ethos* 17 (pp. 68–75). Singapore: Civil Service College.

Thomas, B., Dorling, D., & Smith, G. D. (2010). Inequalities in premature mortality in Britain: Observational study from 1921 to 2007. *BMJ, 341*, c3639.

Thompson, L., Pearce, J., & Barnett, J. R. (2007). Moralising geographies: Stigma, smoking islands and responsible subjects. *Area, 39*(4), 508–517.

Verwei, M., & van den Hoven, M. (2012). Nudges in public health: Paternalism is paramount. *The American Journal of Bioethics, 12*(2), 16–17.

White House. (2015). https://www.whitehouse.gov/ostp/nstc#Committees

Whitehead, M., Howell, R., Jones, R., Lilley, R., & Pykett, J. (2014). *Nudging all over the world: Assessing the global impact of the behavioural sciences on public policy*. Available at: https://changingbehaviours.files.wordpress.com/2014/09/nudgedesignfinal.pdf. Accessed 28 Nov 2017.

Whitehead, M., Jones, R., Lilley, R., Pykett, J., & Howell, R. (2017). *Neuroliberalism. Behavioural government in the twenty-first century*. London: Routledge.

World Bank. (2015). *Mind, society and behaviour: World development report*. Washington, DC: World Bank Group.

World Health Organisation. (1993a). *Social marketing for health*. Geneva: World Health Organisation.

World Health Organisation. (1993b). *Behavioural science learning modules*. Geneva: World Health Organisation.

CHAPTER 5

Who Are the Policymakers and What Are Their Interests?

Holger Strassheim and Kathrin Loer

Abstract Political actors and their interests are significant to policymaking. The chapter gives an overview of the most relevant political actors in public health. But the context of policymaking goes beyond visible political actors. Hence, in a second step the chapter shows which role scientific expertise plays and in what manner it plays this role. The way in which scientific expertise is produced and applied to policymaking by different actors is extremely important in order to understand agenda-setting, the hierarchy of specific policies in public health and ways of implementing those policies in different contexts. This chapter highlights and explains the high degree of complexity that characterises the relationship between policymakers and epistemic authority.

Keywords Policymaking • Scientific expertise • Epistemic authority • Stakeholders

H. Strassheim (✉)
Universität Bielefeld, Bielefeld, Germany
e-mail: holger.strassheim@uni-bielefeld.de

K. Loer
FernUniversität in Hagen, Hagen, Germany
e-mail: kathrin.loer@fernuni-hagen.de

B. Ewert, K. Loer (eds.), *Behavioural Policies for Health Promotion and Disease Prevention*, Palgrave Studies in Public Health Policy Research, https://doi.org/10.1007/978-3-319-98316-5_5

Introduction

Public health is characterised by a high degree of complexity with regard to both the issues involved and how to deal with them—even though, interestingly enough, public health literature identified the 'complexity turn' (Rutter et al. 2017) quite late. It is easy to imagine the huge range of public health issues, ranging from the multitude of communicable diseases (e.g. smallpox, AIDS, HPV, measles) to multifaceted aspects linked with non-communicable diseases (NCDs) such as diabetes, cardiovascular diseases, chronic respiratory diseases, and cancers. For most of these diseases, it is necessary to research their origins, develop strategies for prevention, and implement specific measures (sanitation, vaccination) which may differ according to the societal, environmental, and cultural context. In this sense, it is unsurprising that public health is, by its very nature, closely linked to scientific expertise in order to address major overarching questions: what makes people ill, and what keeps them healthy? The real answers to these questions are to be found in various spheres of medical, biological, epidemiological, psychological, and environmental science (to name but a few). Over the last decade, moreover, we have witnessed the rise of behavioural sciences, which provide insights into human behaviour which can be adapted to public health with varying degrees of ease and success. Generally speaking, decision-making in public health very much depends on this broad spectrum of scientific expertise, and it is important to understand how that expertise is used and applied.

Scientific expertise not only influences policy choices as such, but also to a large extent details of the political agenda-setting and implementation strategies. Furthermore, scientific expertise is not only used by political decision-makers themselves but also by a wide range of stakeholders who play a role in public health. Acknowledging this conceptually, we could distinguish between (generally) independent scientific expertise and scientific advice that has been commissioned by policymakers (government, political parties, interest groups) or by stakeholders (industry, target groups; sometimes disguised as 'independent' expert institutions). But, such a too simplistic dyadic perspective ignores the fact that the transfer of knowledge relies on the ability to adapt scientific knowledge to different spheres of the political process (Fafard and Hoffmann 2018). Besides this adaptability the relationship between policymakers, industry, and science is crucial because it has an impact on agenda-setting, the choice of instrument, the definition of policy targets (see above) and implementation strategies.

Since public health is always closely related to scientific research, it is no surprise that 'evidence-based policymaking' can be identified as (the) major paradigm in this policy area. There are at least three reasons for this: (1) there is a real need for profound knowledge; public health can only be improved if this is done on the basis of a scientific research; (2) evidence-based policy is used strategically to strengthen policymaker's positions, thereby lending them (or at least enabling them to claim) a higher level of legitimacy; and (3) political responsibility could, where necessary and appropriate, be 'up-loaded' to science which means that policymakers use the reference to scientific advice in order to argue that no other option or policy solution is possible (cp. uploading in theories of European Integration). We are aware, of course, that a distinct concept of 'evidence' is lacking and that there can be no guarantee of uncontroversial evidence.

In this chapter, we will not only provide a brief overview of the most relevant policymakers in public health, but we will also analyse ***which role scientific expertise plays and in what manner it plays this role***. The way in which scientific expertise is produced and applied to policymaking by different actors is extremely important in order to understand agenda-setting, the hierarchy of specific policies in public health and ways of implementing those policies in different contexts.

Policymakers in Public Health and the Role of Scientific Expertise

A variety of actors can influence policymaking in public health. Although we probably first think of national governments which have responsibility for their citizen's health status, further reflection may lead us to the international, transnational as well as to regional or local levels. But it does not stop there since many aspects of daily life influence public health but are—at first sight—not (so) closely linked to policymaking. But, these facets are to a large extent shaped by providers of goods and services (market actors), who therefore also play a role in public health. We will then realise that these market actors are linked to policymaking because political decisions can regulate markets in different ways. Hence, market actors also need to be considered when studying policymaking in public health. But with that said, we need to ask how policymakers decide what makes people ill and what keeps them healthy. On what grounds do they make decisions on public health issues? To answer these questions, it is important to get a better understanding of the complex and nuanced role that evidence and expertise play in policymaking.

Considering the political dimension of illness and health, an increasing role can be observed for international and transnational actors. Why is the international and transnational level important in public health policymaking? Many issues in public health are not restricted to national boundaries. In relation to communicable diseases, for instance, there is clearly an urgent need for cooperation and coordination in order to implement international and transnational strategies: epidemics, for example, do not stop at political borders. Governments can only fight epidemics effectively if they cooperate with local actors, neighbouring governments and usually also with international organisations (e.g. explained in the context of new 'governance approaches' Leach et al. 2010). Furthermore, vaccines are developed by multinational companies (MNCs) and have to be distributed internationally to be economically feasible for manufacturers. Consequently, MNCs have an interest in inter- and transnational cooperation and seek to gain a foothold in vaccination policy. Similarly, policymakers rely on the research activities of pharmaceutical companies, which often take on the economic risks involved in the development of vaccines. As with communicable diseases, we see that NCDs are not limited to national contexts and also lead to cross-border interdependencies: NCDs are very often the result of unhealthy lifestyles and habits that emerge and proliferate in many countries simultaneously, not least because of similar lifestyle patterns and the consumption of similar products, which are successfully marketed in capitalist societies nearly all over the world. To gauge all these developments (in NCDs and CDs) and to cope with their sheer complexity, political actors often use quantification through numbers and scales as a starting-point for decision-making procedures, for example, to reduce complexity. Numbers and scales are relevant in both spheres of public health (CDs and NCDs) in three ways: first, in order to classify a public health issue; second, to observe developments; and third, to monitor the effects of public health policies.

Numbers and scales are especially useful when considering the social determinants of health. With regard to this sphere of public health, one might argue that the local or regional levels are decisive or even more important than the international and transnational contexts. There is no doubt that the social determinants of people's health are at first glance strongly influenced by a person's immediate physical environment and that this is (normally) local or regional in scope. But in this respect, too, we can identify a significant role for international and transnational actors (e.g. WHO, OECD) who not only develop programmes for intervening in regional health contexts, initiate mutual learning (policy-learning) or transfer policies between countries (Kickbusch 2003), but also provide and disseminate the numbers and scales by which public health is quantified (for a suggestion to develop good practice for health statistic see Murray 2007). Furthermore, many stakeholders have, directly and indirectly, some influence on social determinants since their products play a role in healthy or unhealthy habits and lifestyles. Thus, stakeholders become the addressees of public health policies where these influences can be measured (e.g. a correlation between the consumption of a certain product and the prevalence of a certain disease). A preliminary conclusion might be that public health problems involve political actors which actually and directly decide on different levels of policymaking (from local/regional to international level). But the character of public health problems also leads to the conclusion that a multitude of actors are involved, all of which are linked and interdependent, so that actors sometimes affect or rely on each other (shown, e.g. from the perspective of international relations in Youde 2012 and Davies 2010). To deal with such complexity, numbers and scales (often) seem to be the means of choice. Scientific research in public health can provide common ground for cooperation between actors, their relationships, and interdependencies, as much as for policymaking that is based on 'evidence'—but linking scientific knowledge and public health policymaking is a challenging and risky task.

The scientific dimension adds even more complexity to the field of public health. A vast number of studies inform us of correlations between specific factors and poor health or risks to health. With regard to that political science grapples with important questions (e.g. Hawkins and Parkurst 2016): Who decides which studies are reliable in relation to a certain issue in public health policymaking? Who decides on the indicators used to classify a status as a 'problem'? How can policymakers make use of public health research in the best way possible? And how can they do so without unintentionally being influenced in a certain direction? Public health scholars often complain about the 'research-policy gap' (Oliver et al. 2014) and there seems to be a transfer problem when it comes to public health. One solution could be to provide public policy with the best and most valid scientific evidence while leaving decisions to policy makers. Many authors, however, argue that this is an idealistic view of the complex and intricate relationship between science and policy. The empirical example of International Life Science Institute (ILSI) in this chapter will address these interlinkages and illustrate how insisting on the separation of science and policy may have consequences such as a microfixation in the case of behavioural public policy promoted by ILSI.

Scientific knowledge may influence public health policymaking in a specific direction, even though it has (most likely) departed from the acceptable research norms. In such cases, what is presented as scientific knowledge in fact lacks objectivity and is transformed into a kind of lobbying activity. Potentially, this transformation is not explicitly disclosed in such cases, and we see institutions emerge that conceal their true sponsors, motives, and the ulterior objectives of their research activities (see section "International Life Science Institute"). The empirical example in this chapter will address these observations (cp. Cairney 2016) and illustrate how scientific research is produced by stakeholders and channelled into public health policymaking.

Any discussion of policymakers and stakeholders in public health requires greater specificity. Since we have started from a broad understanding of policymakers, we will focus not only on elected representatives or international organisations, but we will also refer to the potential addressees of public health policy who may have an interest in co-creating policies. This applies particularly to those stakeholders that offer products (or sometimes services) which affect people's health directly or indirectly. It is easy to imagine a range of legally available products that have a direct and adverse effect on health if consumed regularly or above a certain dosage (e.g. alcohol, sugar). Several other factors indirectly affect people's health—such as low standards of hygiene in hospitals or outpatient clinics; the contamination of consumer goods (e.g. dioxin contaminated eggs in Germany.); poor working conditions which lead to injuries and/or mental stress; limited, opaque, or overly complex information regarding the risks associated with products, whether technical risks or the risk of misuse, and so the list continues. When governments consider responding to these risks with legislation or regulations in order to safeguard or improve public health, a range of actors may be addressed, including those who would see their business activities restricted. In such situations, stakeholders search for ways of influencing policymaking in order to preserve their market (share), prevent stricter regulation or establish new products and services in the way that they prefer. Particularly large players (MNCs, etc.) very often refer to scientific research, which they seek to transfer into policymaking. They not only use this scientific 'support' to refute the case for particular forms of regulation, but also actively use 'expertise' to co-create policies. Meanwhile we can observe how stakeholders develop networks or agency structures. These institutions function as independent actors, as intermediaries which are meant to provide policymakers with background information on a specific topic or field (we will return to this with the example of the ILSI in section "International Life Science Institute").

From a conceptual perspective, it is worth looking very closely not only at such intermediaries but also at stakeholders. This quite new structure of intermediaries is part of a bigger picture that shows the links between stakeholders and policymakers. Stakeholders still engage in 'traditional' lobbying on matters that concern public health issues at various policy-levels. During the last decade, these lobbying activities have been intensified whenever someone called for 'fighting obesity'. Although obesity has been the subject of extensive discussion, it touches on many other fields of policymaking: agricultural policy, urban policy, rural policy, labour market policy, education policy, economic policy, and social policy—to name a few of the most relevant policy areas. Elected politicians, administrative staff at the national and international levels, representatives in international organisations (e.g. WHO) are—at least potentially—the objects of lobbying activities from many different directions. Comprehensive studies, for example, the seminal work of Nestle (Nestle 2002), show a strong alliance between farmers who produce sugar cane or beet and producers of processed food, whose interests would contrast with paediatricians concerned about the future health and well-being of overweight and obese children, health insurance companies who must cover the costs of treatments for NCDs caused by excess weight or obesity, and possibly employers who have already detected signs of falling productivity among those suffering from these NCDs. However, this small example indicates one major problem in public health policymaking: there is a huge power imbalance between stakeholders. On the one hand, there are those who have the wherewithal to shape the political agenda, or pursue a common purpose that can easily be consolidated. On the other hand, we see a potentially large but diverse group of actors, often without financial power and resources, and often with a less coherent set of motives and aims.

As we have seen, policymakers in public health are driven by a range of factors and with a range of objectives. It is important to consider the political and scientific dimensions of policymaking that produce a certain kind of 'expertise'. Expertise generally shifts between science and politics and should not be confused with science. We understand expertise as knowledge that is indeed valid in terms of scientific standards, but at the same time is politically relevant. The following section uses the example of the industry-founded ILSI that has become a major proponent of evidence-based policy and behavioural approaches in public health. It serves as illustration for three different perceptions of expertise in public health: Some argue that the global proliferation of expert organisations is the result of a large-scale scientisation of global public health ('scientizing global public health'). Others maintain, that in contrast, industry-founded expert organisation such as ILSI have their ways of spinning science and should be understood as a symptom of the commercialisation and politicisation of science ('commercialising and politicising science'). Both perspectives implicitly or explicitly insist on separating science from politics. A third group of authors argue that, paradoxically, by insisting on this separation, advocators of pure science may unknowingly be helping to create opportunities for the hidden influence of industries and interest groups. They do not deny the manipulation of science for political and industrial purposes. Yet, they draw the attention to a scientistic obsession with consensual knowledge and pure facts, which could help to shift attention away from the necessary practices of selection, valuation and implicit 'mobilization of bias' (Schattschneider 1961) that are inextricably intertwined with the operations of expertise at the boundaries between science and policy ('knowing and governing health policy'). In the case of behavioural public policy, this could lead to a problematic interlinkage between the ever-increasing search for scientific rigidity with a more or less unquestioned shift from the structural dimension of health problems to the level of the individual.

International Life Science Institute[1]

In 1978, six large food, chemical, and drug companies—Coca-Cola, Pepsi-Cola, Heinz, Kraft Foods (owned by Philip Morris), General Foods, and Procter & Gamble—founded the International Life Science Institute, also known as ILSI. Based in Washington D.C., ILSI became a worldwide organisation with 17 regional and country-specific branches including a focal point in China, the ILSI Health and Environmental Sciences Institute, the ILSI Research Foundation, and 'One ILSI', a transnational

[1]The empirical research carried out for this chapter by Holger Strassheim was supported by the Franco-German Research Program of the Humanities and Social Sciences 'Changing Societies' at the Berlin Social Science Center (WZB) and the Fondation maison des sciences de l'homme (FMSH) in Paris. Thanks are extended to the other authors of this volume and to Nastasja Rostalski for valuable research assistance.

networking programme that encourages collaborative research between ILSI entities across policy areas such as food and water safety, risk assessment, nutrition, and agricultural sustainability.

ILSI can be seen as a paradigmatic example of multiple and seemingly contradictory dynamics in global public health: as a non-profit organisation 'whose mission is to provide science that improves human health and well-being' by bringing together 'scientists from geographically diverse regions of the world' (ILSI 2018a), the organisation represents the large-scale scientisation of public policy as reflected in the increase in international and transnational knowledge actors (Zapp 2018). As an industry foundation with more than 400 companies as paying members, however, ILSI is seen by its critics as an attempt to infiltrate science and exert influence on global public health and food policy in the name of commercial interests (Grimm 2017). In many ways, ILSI seems to incorporate both tendencies: the scientisation of public health and public policy in general; and the politico-economic instrumentalisation of science. It is a multifaceted organisation which illustrates how politics and expertise have become intertwined under the conditions of the 'post-national constellation' (Strassheim 2017b).

Scientising Global Public Health

In 1917, Max Weber famously argued in his lecture on 'Science as Vocation' that science had become a rationalising force, disenchanting the world and driven by the belief that 'one could in principle master everything through calculation' (Weber 2015 [1917], 13). According to Weber, the principles of science pervade all features of modern society by setting standards, establishing rational bureaucracies, developing technologies, controlling experience by experiments, governing by knowledge—and forcing each and every person to make sense of his or her actions without resorting to references to higher powers. In the tradition of Weber's classic assumptions about the rationalisation of the world, more recent research argues that there is indeed a global trend towards formal organisation, standardisation, and scientisation across a very diverse range of social contexts (Drori et al. 2003; Zapp 2018).

Especially in globalised and highly complex policy areas such as public health, the number of intergovernmental organisations (IGOs), international research institutes (IRIs) and nongovernmental organisations (INGOs) has risen dramatically (Zapp 2018): Over the past 100 years, the number of IGOs has increased from 37 in the early 20th century to 7710 today; similarly, the number of INGOs has risen from 200 before the First World War to more than 60,000 organisations today. More importantly, the scientific output of these organisations has expanded considerably with organisations in both energy policy and public health as top producers of research publications (Zapp 2018, 14). Since the early 2000s, they have enlarged their annual scientific output. Based on a sample of more than 1300 international organisations, Zapp (2018) shows that in health-related areas, IGOs, INGOs, and IRIs have published over 24,000 papers, more than in any other policy area (except for energy with roughly 30,000 publications). The World Health Organisation is among the top ten producers of research (Zapp 2018, 16). Moreover, by promoting cross-organisational collaboration, international organisations both create and multiply venues for producing scientific knowledge in the international and transnational spheres. Beyond the university as the 'locus classicus' of research, international organisations 'have shifted from regulative and normative authority through treaties and naming and shaming to a more cognitive kind of authority represented in their accumulation of rationalized knowledge' (Zapp 2018, 21). The increasing density of networks among academic researchers, private companies, governments, and civil society organisations changes the ways in which expertise and scientific knowledge are translated into public policies.

These observations are mirrored by what has become a broad consensus across multiple research fields in public policy studies, international relations, and political sociology (Quack 2016; Zürn et al. 2012; Fischer 2009; Strassheim 2015): in a world of unprecedented cross-border communication, more and more collective actors are struggling for both political and epistemic authority, that is, for acceptance as being competent to validate and justify knowledge claims ('epistemic authority') and of being capable of making these knowledge claims relevant to the collective ordering and evaluating of society ('political authority'). Some argue that these networks are part of a 'global agora', a more or less open marketplace of ideas and interaction at the private-policy nexus (Stone 2012). Others are more sceptical, assuming that the ongoing fragmentation and contestation of authority may strengthen the hand of 'unelected' actors that do not draw on democratic sources of legitimacy (such as central banks, independent agencies, INGOs, and IRIs), while reducing the power of democratically legitimate institutions (Vibert 2007; Zürn 2017; Strassheim 2015).

ILSI is a case in point. In the 40 years of its existence, it has remained largely unknown to the public but, at the same time, has played an increasingly prominent role in the global politics of public health, food safety, and sustainability (Grimm 2017, 14; Hendrickx 2017; Demortain 2009; Greenhalgh 2016). ILSI's board of trustees is composed of members of transnational corporations such as Nestlé, Procter & Gamble, Pepsi, Danone, and Monsanto and at least 50 percent of public sector members from universities, academia, and research agencies in the United States, United Kingdom, Japan, Australia, Germany, Taiwan, Brazil, the Netherlands, Mexico, Canada, India, France, Korea, and Switzerland. Among its members, it lists over 400 multinational companies that provide roughly two-thirds of its financial support (ILSI 2016a). To this date, ILSI has established 16 branches based in Argentina, Brazil, Europe, India, Japan, Korea, Latin America, Mesoamerica, Mexico, the Middle East, North America, North Andean, South Africa, Southeast Asia, Taiwan, and a 'focal point' in China.

ILSI publicises the fact that it 'believes its science—as part of the larger body of scientific information—helps industries make safer, healthier products and helps governments, civil society organisations, and individual health professionals provide effective and practical guidance to promote safety, health, and well-being' (ILSI 2018a). To achieve these goals, ILSI has defined four 'thematic areas' that capture the core of ILSI's activities: food and water safety; nutrition and health; risk science and toxicology; sustainable agriculture and nutrition security. Advocacy, as the ILSI's code of ethics states, 'is strictly limited to the promotion of the use of evidence-based science as an aid in decision-making' (ILSI 2016b). As an international non-profit research organisation, ILSI has become one of the strongest proponents of the global 'evidence-based policy' movement (Strassheim 2017b), arguing that 'decisions affecting public health and safety are based on good science' (ILSI 2016c). This insistence on the essential role of evidence and science in public policy is also reflected in ILSI's research centres, institutes, and programmes. The ILSI Research Foundation, formed in 1984, has established four 'centres of excellence': the Center for Environmental Risk Assessment, the Center for Integrated Modeling of Sustainable Agriculture & Nutrition Security, the Center for Risk Science Innovation and Application, and the Center for Safety Assessment of Food and Feed. These different sub-organisations provide databases such as the 'GM Crop Database' or the 'ILSI Crop Composition Database', develop methods of risk evaluation and decision-making and disseminate approaches for the treatment of health issues such as obesity, malnutrition, and so on. In 1989, ILSI established the Health and Environmental Sciences Institute (HESI) as a global branch 'to advance the understanding of scientific issues related to human health, toxicology, risk assessment, and the environment'. In 2002, HESI was recognised by the US government as a non-profit, tax exempt organisation, and it became independent in 2018 as a global organisation with more than 200 members including academic institutions, government agencies, corporations, consultants, and other public sector organisations.

Based on this overview, ILSI seems to be the prototypical global non-profit research actor, carrying out its activities at the interface of science, politics, and industry, and providing scientific data and regulatory tools across a broad spectrum of issues relating to global health, food, and the environment. It is not a network but, more accurately, a 'meta-organisation' (Ahrne and Brunsson 2008), which manages inter-organisational relationships, incorporates institutes and research programmes, and creates new and independent organisational entities such as HESI—all in the name of promoting 'evidence-based policy'. However, if we only view ILSI from the perspective of the scientisation of public policy, we are missing the flip side of this coin: the politicisation and commercialisation of science.

Commercialising and Politicising Science

ILSI's membership list reads like the 'Who's Who' of Big Food and Big Health. As Grimm (2017, 15) argues, 'ILSI is an army of Big Food, a powerful association of the big boys, of those companies which dominate the global food supply with increasing power [...]'. When ILSI was created in 1978, one of its founding fathers, Alex Malaspina, a leading strategist and 'vice-director' of Coca-Cola, was said to have been motivated by rumours about the toxicity of caffeine; by creating ILSI, the story goes, he was hoping for an instrument to counter these rumours based on science (Hendrickx 2017). It is a common narrative: the 'spinning of science' in the name of corporate interests (Gilliam 2017, 114): 'What the public doesn't know is that behind the scenes, corporations are often funding and collaborating closely with these very same professors and other professionals who tout propaganda that serves industry interests. It's all part of a strategy of spin that has been used by the tobacco industry, the soft drink industry, pharmaceuticals, and, of course, agriculture'.

In 2003, *The Guardian* published an article saying that the WHO had been 'infiltrated by food industry' and criticising the 'easy movements' of experts between universities, multinational industries, and government research institutes (Boseley 2003). According to a confidential report obtained by *The Guardian*, ILSI had 'positioned its experts and expertise across the whole spectrum of food and tobacco policies: at conferences, on FAO/WHO food policy committees and within WHO, and with monographs, journals and technical briefs'. Similarly, the European Food Safety Authority (EFSA) has always been criticised for its close ties to ILSI (Grimm 2017). In 2012, Diána Bánáti, the chair of the EFSA advisory board and at the same time a board member at ILSI, had to resign from her position at EFSA, only to become ILSI's scientific director. The close links between ILSI and EFSA became especially apparent in the case of Aspartame, a sweeter used as replacement for sugar (Grimm 2017, 18–22). While scientific studies were presenting increasing evidence that Aspartame may have serious side-effects including acute disorders, headaches, brain damages, and even brain tumours, the EFSA saw no reason to reconsider its earlier approval of the substance. The EFSA expert panel, which re-evaluated Aspartame in 2009 and decided that is was harmless, consisted of several experts who also served in ILSI committees or even worked as representatives of active ILSI member corporations including the Aspartame corporation Ajinomoto, Aspartame customer Coca-Cola, and the Danish sweetener suppliers Danisco (Grimm 2017, 21).

Given the multiple instances in which regulatory bodies and public health organisations are interwoven with meta-organisations such as ILSI, we might indeed come to the more sceptical conclusion that the scientisation of public policy has, in fact, been accompanied and even undermined by the rapid commercialisation and political instrumentalisation of science (Clapp and Scrinis 2017; Zapp 2018; Nestle 2002). By focusing on the scientific properties of food and pharmaceuticals, big firms enhance their legitimacy to intervene in policy and governance contexts. Using expertise to open doors, private-sector actors engage in advisory bodies, committees, and expert panels, raising their voice in the name of science to shape discussions, to draw attention away from wider health and food problems caused by their own activities and even to present themselves and their products as the solution. Policymakers, in turn, borrow the epistemic authority of industry experts to legitimise political decisions and to gain leverage in highly complex policy areas. 'Evidence-based policy making', it seems, has become 'policy- and profit-based evidence making' (Strassheim and Kettunen 2014). Almost 100 years ago, Weber warned us that the only person who could maintain a 'relative immunity' to the rationalising force of knowledge was the 'capitalist entrepreneur' (Weber 1978 [1922]).

Knowing and Governing Health Policy

The case of ILSI, however, may illuminate an even more complex dimension beyond the linear opposition between scientisation and commercialisation, between value-free science and interest-driven decision-making. The notion that scientifically approved facts are value-free, which are then disregarded or, worse, ideologically 'polluted' when they cross the boundary into the zone of politico-administrative procedures may be overly simplistic. The frequent equation of expertise with science should be treated with caution. Experts are always already boundary workers. More often than not, policy-relevant facts are the result of an intensive and complex struggle for political and epistemic authority on both sides—expertise as well as policy. This applies particularly where science and policy are closely interlinked and the guidelines for validating knowledge are highly contested. Expert organisations in complex areas such as health policy are already operating in the zone of intertwinement between science and policy, where expert authority is collectively defined, indicators and their interpretation have to be negotiated, insiders are separated from outsiders and credibility is always 'on the line' (Gieryn 1998).

Paradoxically, by insisting on separating expertise from political considerations, advocators of the 'linearity-autonomy model of science for policy' (Jasanoff 2011) may even be helping to create opportunities for the hidden dominance of political and commercial interests. Debates regarding public values, the desirability of policy solutions, the regulation of risks, or the anticipation of future challenges may easily be suspended in the quest for science-based policy. This is not to deny the influence of corporate power, the spinning of science, the funnelling of industry messages by selected experts, the manipulation of studies, the gaming, cheating, and cherry-picking. It is beyond doubt that these practices exist and they are characteristic of policy areas such as public health (Gilliam 2017). Yet the deeper or, in the words of Rittel and Webber (Rittel and Webber 1973), the truly 'wicked' problem could be the technocratic fixation on consensual knowledge and scientific facts, which helps to shift attention away from the underlying constructions of necessity, the 'governance by numbers' and the politics of standardising and structuring the ways of both knowing and governing health policy (Demortain 2009; Hendrickx 2017).

One of the most telling examples is that of the creation of an NCD labelled as 'obesity' in China (for the following see Greenhalgh 2016). It is closely linked to ILSI, and especially its Focal Point China, an entity dedicated to providing science-based advice and 'scientific tools' to the Ministry of Health in China. As early as 1999, ILSI had placed obesity on its list of core issues relevant for all sectors. With the help of pharmaceuticals like Knoll and Roche the worldwide body mass index (BMI) cut-off standards for obesity and excess weight were defined, and guidelines for managing obesity were developed. Taking the WHO standards of obesity science as the gold standard, experts from the International Obesity Task Force (IOTF) started to research the problem in China, a country that had traditionally taken a favourable view of excess body weight as a sign of prosperity. This traditional image was challenged when the experts from IOTF in cooperation with ILSI Focal Point China started to discuss China-specific cut-off points for obesity based on evidence on Chinese and Asian bodies. Given these studies, the expert committee proposed China-specific cut-offs of 24 and 28 for overweight and obesity, respectively (compared to the standards for Western countries adopted by the WHO in 1998 with a BMI of 25 as the cut-off for excess weight and 30 for obesity). This was the beginning of the obesity crisis in China, apparently requiring an urgent strategy for education and lifestyle changes—and providing an opportunity for companies such as Coca-Cola to become a regular member of ILSI China and to advise the Chinese government on nutrition and unhealthy foods. As this example shows, it is not the instrumentalisation of science by corporate interests, but the uninhibited quest for purely science-based cut-off points that has restructured this policy area, sparking off a health crisis and paving the way for corporate influence on public health (Greenhalgh 2016, 505).

In line with these and other activities, ILSI has defined 'Consumer Behaviour Activities' as a key priority area for the future. The subject of 'Nudging and Sustainable Changes Towards Healthier Food Choices' has already been developed by an ILSI expert group into a 'New Activity Proposal', assessing evidence 'on if and when nudging can lead to long-term behavioural changes' (ILSI 2018b). Over the past decade, behavioural strategies have become influential, especially in health and consumer policy, by combining the epistemic authority of experimental studies with the relevance of a policy claiming to achieve a significant impact with small regulatory interventions (Strassheim 2017a)—a political strategy for avoiding coercive instruments (see Chap. 3 in this book). Again, this is not so much about the commercialisation of science or the manipulation of expertise. Behavioural health policies may, however, lead to the combination of the search for scientific rigidity with a more or less unquestioned shift from the structural dimension of health problems to the level of the individual. Instead of designing laws and regulations that focus on the market forces that shape the health environment or constraining industry's control over health policy, randomised controlled trials on changing individual behaviour have become the 'gold standard' for informing public policy. For the food and health industry, no manipulation is needed when the most robust evidence is to be found at the micro-level, where regulatory restrictions would also be the least intrusive in relation to commercial interests.

Conclusion

This chapter highlights the high degree of complexity that characterises the relationship between policymakers and epistemic authority. Given the multiplicity of actors at different levels of global public health, it would be too simplistic to assume one-way lobbying activities, from industry to policymakers. Rather, we see multiple and sometimes contradictory dynamics.

Firstly, scientific expertise has entered the relationship between market actors and policymakers. In line with Weber's assumptions concerning the rationalisation and scientisation of the world, the number of international expert organisations has expanded dramatically over the past 100 years. As recent research shows, the scientific output of these organisations has also expanded, with organisations in public health among top producers of research publications. By promoting cross-organisational collaboration, there has been a proliferation in venues for the production of scientific knowledge in the international and transnational sphere. ILSI has become one of the strongest proponents of the global 'evidence-based policy' movement, providing not only data but also standards and guidelines to organisations of regulatory science in public health, nutrition, and sustainability by promoting its research centres, institutes, and science programmes.

Secondly, given the dominance of multinational corporations in organisations such as ILSI, one might conclude that the scientisation of public policy is, in fact, being accompanied and undermined by the rapid commercialisation and political instrumentalisation of science. Using expertise as a way of opening doors, large corporations engage with advisory bodies, committees, and expert panels to frame discussions in the name of science, to draw attention away from structural health and food problems caused by their own market activities and even to present themselves and their products as solutions. Policymakers, in turn, draw on the epistemic authority of industry experts to legitimise their political decisions.

Thirdly, the case of ILSI illustrates an even more complex dimension beyond the simple notion that facts are value-free, and only become ideologically 'polluted' when they cross the boundary into politics. Where science and policy are closely interlinked and the guidelines for validating knowledge are highly contested, policy-relevant facts are the result of an intensive and complex struggle. Expert organisations in globalised domains such as health policy are already operating in the zone of intertwinement between science and policy. By insisting on separating expertise from political considerations, advocates of the linear mode of policy advice ignore this political dimension of expertise and knowledge production. Here, the problem is not so much the manipulation of science for commercial purposes but a fixation on objective knowledge and scientific facts. Interestingly enough, the development of institutions such as ILSI and stakeholder's activities to strengthen certain forms of expertise and transfer these into policymaking goes hand in hand with a development described in all chapters of this book: policymaking in public health is increasingly characterised by the shift from the structural dimension of health problems to the individual level. More often than not, structural problems and social inequalities involved in public health and food are being neglected in the name of 'evidence-based policy'.

References

Ahrne, G., & Brunsson, N. (2008). *Meta-organizations.* Cheltenham/Northampton: Edward Elgar.

Boseley, S. (2003). *WHO 'Infiltrated by food industry'*. Available at: https://www.theguardian.com/uk/2003/jan/09/foodanddrink. Last accessed 4 Mar 2018.

Cairney, P. (2016). *The politics of evidence-based policy making.* London: Palgrave Macmillan.

Clapp, J., & Scrinis, G. (2017). Big food, nutritionism, and corporate power. *Globalizations, 14*(4), 578–595.

Davies, S. (2010). *Global politics of health*. Cambridge/Malden: Polity Press.
Demortain, D. (2009). Legitimation by standards: Transnational experts, the European Commission and regulation of novel foods. *Sociologie du travail, 51S*, e104–e116.
Drori, G. S., Meyer, J. W., Ramirez, F. O., et al. (2003). *Science in the modern world polity. Institutionalization and globalization*. Stanford: Stanford University Press.
Fafard, P., & Hoffman, S. (2018). Rethinking knowledge translation for public health policy. *Evidence & Policy: A Journal of Research, Debate and Practice*. Retrieved from http://www.ingentaconnect.com/content/tpp/ep/pre-prints/content-ppevidpol1700028r3
Fischer, F. (2009). *Democracy & expertise. Reorienting policy inquiry*. Oxford: Oxford University Press.
Gieryn, T. F. (1998). *Cultural boundaries of science. Credibility on the line*. Chicago/London: University of Chicago.
Gilliam, C. (2017). *Whitewash. The story of a weed killer, cancer, and the corruption of science*. Washington, DC: Island Press.
Greenhalgh, S. (2016). Neoliberal science, Chinese style: Making and managing the 'obesity epidemic'. *Social Studies of Science, 46*(4), 485–510.
Grimm, H.-U. (2017). Information-domination in the European food industry: Focus on Germany. In G. Steier & K. K. Patel (Eds.), *International food law and policy* (pp. 3–30). Cham: Springer.
Hawkins, B., & Parkhurst, J. (2016). The 'good governance' of evidence in health policy. *Evidence & Policy: A Journal of Research, Debate and Practice, 12*(4), 575–592.
Hendrickx, K. (2017). Working imagination along the food-drug divide. In G. Verschraegen, F. Vandermoere, L. Braeckmans, et al. (Eds.), *Imagined futures in science, technology, and society*. Oxon/New York: Routledge.
ILSI. (2016a). *2015 Member and Supporting Companies*. Available at: http://ilsi.org/wp-content/uploads/2016/01/Members.pdf. Last accessed 3 Mar 2018.
ILSI. (2016b). *Code of ethics and organizational standards of conduct*. Available at: http://ilsi.org/wp-content/uploads/2016/05/ILSICodeofEthicsSofC2009.pdf. Last accessed 3 Mar 2018.
ILSI. (2016c). *The role and activities of ILSI Europe*. Available at: http://ilsi.org/europe/wp-content/uploads/sites/3/2016/05/ILSI-FREQUENTLY-ASKED-QUESTIONS.pdf. Last accessed 3 Mar 2018.
ILSI. (2018a). *Mission and operating principles*. Available at: http://ilsi.org/about/mission/
ILSI. (2018b). *Status of the new activity on 'consumer behaviour determinants'*. Available at: http://ilsi.eu/emerging-issues/. Last accessed 3 Mar 2018.

Jasanoff, S. (2011). Quality control and peer review in advisory science. In J. Lentsch & P. Weingart (Eds.), *The politics of scientific advice. Institutional design for quality assurance* (pp. 19–35). Cambridge/New York/Melbourne: Cambridge University Press.

Kickbusch, I. (2003). The contribution of the World Health Organization to a new public health and health promotion. *American Journal of Public Health, 93*(3), 383–388.

Leach, M., Scoones, I., & Stirling, A. (2010). Governing epidemics in an age of complexity: Narratives, politics and pathways to sustainability. *Global Environmental Change, 20*(3), 369–377.

Murray, C. J. (2007). Towards good practice for health statistics: Lessons from the Millennium Development Goal health indicators. *The Lancet, 369*(9564), 862–873.

Nestle, M. (2002). *Food politics: How the food industry influences nutrition and health* (Revised ed.). Berkeley: University of California Press.

Oliver, K., Innvar, S., Lorenc, T., Woodman, J., & Thomas, J. (2014). A systematic review of barriers to and facilitators of the use of evidence by policymakers. *BMC Health Services Research, 14*(1), 2.

Quack, S. (2016). Expertise and authority in transnational governance. In R. Cotterrell & M. Del Mar (Eds.), *Authority in transnational legal theory. Theorising across disciplines*. Cheltenham/Northampton: Edward Elgar.

Rittel, H. W. J., & Webber, M. M. (1973). Dilemmas in a general theory of planning. *Policy Sciences, 4*(2), 155–169.

Rutter, H., Savona, N., Glonti, K., Bibby, J., Cummins, S., Finegood, D. T., et al. (2017). The need for a complex systems model of evidence for public health. *The Lancet, 390*(10112), 2602–2604.

Schattschneider, E. E. (1961). *The semisovereign people, A realist's view of democracy in America*. New York: Holt Rinehart and Winston.

Stone, D. (2012). *Knowledge actors and transnational governance: The private-public policy Nexus in the global Agora*. London: Palgrave Macmillan.

Strassheim, H. (2015). Politics and policy expertise: Towards a political epistemology. In F. Fischer, D. Torgerson, A. Durnová, et al. (Eds.), *Handbook of critical policy studies* (pp. 319–340). Cheltenham/Northampton: Edward Elgar.

Strassheim, H. (2017a). Behavioural expertise and regulatory power in Europe. In M. Lee, A. de Ruiter, & M. Weimer (Eds.), *Regulating risks in the European Union* (pp. 143–163). Oxford: Hart.

Strassheim, H. (2017b). Trends towards evidence-based policy formulation. In M. Howlett & I. Mukherjee (Eds.), *Handbook of policy formulation* (pp. 504–521). Cheltenham/Northampton: Edward Elgar.

Strassheim, H., & Kettunen, P. (2014). When does evidence-based policy turn into policy-based evidence? Configurations, contexts and mechanisms. *Evidence & Policy, 10*(2), 259–277.

Vibert, F. (2007). *The rise of the unelected: Democracy and the new separation of powers*. Cambridge: Cambridge University Press.
Weber, M. (1978 [1922]). *Economy and society. An outline of interpretive sociology* (G. Roth & C. Wittich, Eds.). Berkeley/Los Angeles/London: University of California Press.
Weber, M. (2015 [1917]). Science as a vocation. In P. Lassmann, I. Velody, & H. Martins (Eds.), *Max Weber's 'Science as a vocation'*. London/New York: Routledge.
Youde, J. R. (2012). *Global health governance*. Cambridge/Malden: Polity Press.
Zapp, M. (2018). The scientization of the world polity: International organizations and the production of scientific knowledge, 1950–2015. *International Sociology, 33*(1), 3–26.
Zürn, M. (2017). From constitutional rule to loosely coupled spheres of liquid authority: A reflexive approach. *International Theory, 9*(2), 261–285.
Zürn, M., Binder, M., & Ecker-Ehrhardt, M. (2012). International authority and its politicization. *International Theory – A Journal of International Politics, Law and Philosophy, 4*(1), 69–106.

CHAPTER 6

Conclusion: Towards a Behaviourally Informed Health Citizenship

Benjamin Ewert and Kathrin Loer

Abstract The conclusion recapitulates main findings concerning policymaking in public health in the light of the behavioural turn. First, the huge potential that behavioural policies could hold, if they are combined with classic instruments for health promotion, will be emphasised. Second, implications of the rise of behavioural health policies for the concept of health citizenship and state-citizen relations are discussed. By suggesting the concept of a 'behaviourally informed health citizenship', it will be argued that a reconciliation between citizenship and behavioural governance is feasible.

Keywords Health promotion • Social determinants of health • Behavioural interventions • Health nudges • Policymaking • Citizenship

B. Ewert
FernUniversität in Hagen, Hagen, Germany
e-mail: benjamin.ewert@fernuni-hagen.de

K. Loer (✉)
FernUniversität in Hagen, Hagen, Germany
e-mail: kathrin.loer@fernuni-hagen.de

B. Ewert, K. Loer (eds.), *Behavioural Policies for Health Promotion and Disease Prevention*, Palgrave Studies in Public Health Policy Research, https://doi.org/10.1007/978-3-319-98316-5_6

Conclusion

The objective of this book, as set out in Chap. 1, has been to provide the reader with a better understanding of the challenges of policymaking in public health in the light of current behavioural policies. As we arrive at the final chapter of the book, it is time to take stock of our main findings concerning the primary research question. We will proceed in two steps. First, we will answer the question of what kind of public health policy we may be heading for in the years to come. Future health policy will be dominated by the spread of non-communicable diseases (NCDs) which will pose severely challenges for national health systems and economies (if they do not already). Second, we will turn to a major issue in this book and develop this even further: what are the implications of the rise of behavioural health policies for the concept of health citizenship and state-citizen relations? Our answer to this question is the quest for a 'behaviourally informed concept of citizenship'.

Policymaking in Public Health in the Light of the Behavioural Turn

Finding appropriate solutions to today's most pressing public health problems seems to be a Sisyphean task because of the crucial insight that 'complex problems require complex solutions' (de Leeuw and Peters 2014, 987) such as *Health in All Policies* (HiAP). In this vein, the infamous spaghetti diagram illustrating the potential factors involved in obesity[1] exemplifies perfectly the multiplicity of factors that influence obesity and their many interconnections (Butland et al. 2007). De Leeuw and Peters (2014, 990) point a way *out of the spaghetti* by demonstrating that in HiAP practices 'complexity can be dealt with systematically'. However, in order to contain—or at least control—the obesity epidemic, there is 'neither a distinct problem-solution-nexus nor a strict correlation between issues/problems and policy instruments' (Chap. 3). However, while public health, as a scientific discipline, has been traditionally fairly good at producing evidence on the 'causes of the causes' (Marmot 2005, 1101) of

[1] Unfortunately, the diagram cannot be printed in a reader-friendly way in this book. An interactive learning tool that impressively explains the complexity of obesity is available online via http://www.shiftn.com/obesity/Full-Map.html.

diseases and illness, it has only recently started to advance our collective knowledge and expertise on policymaking in public health (Clavier and de Leeuw 2013)—that is to say, to engage itself with the policy process and the choice of political instruments in order to achieve improvements in public health (Chap. 3). Redirecting the focus of public health onto the process of policymaking could be disappointing: the overwhelming evidence on the impact of the social determinants of health is not automatically translated into comprehensive policy concepts for health promotion, such as the settings approach (Dooris 2009). This is due to the inherent dynamics of policymaking processes and the dominant paradigm of policies that primarily focus on individual lifestyles.

As set out in this book, the recent 'behavioural turn' (Crawshaw 2013) in public health adds an additional layer to the policymaking process, that is, policy instruments are being affected by a 'behavioural spin' (Chap. 3), which may at first sight appear to be a silver lining. However, behaviourally informed policies may also reinforce the current paradigm that interventions tend to address the individual level rather than tackling structural problems. In contrast to this empirical observation, we would like to emphasise the huge potential that behavioural policies could hold, particularly if they are combined with classic instruments for health promotion. Hence, in their current form, most behaviourally informed policies (i.e. policy instruments and instrument mixes influenced by the behavioural spin) emphasise individual responsibility for health by promoting individual self-regulation. At the same time, behavioural policies tend 'to downplay other significant drivers of public health and health inequalities' (Chap. 4). So far, behavioural interventions seem merely to be a contemporary modification of the long-standing tradition of health promotion strategies, which fit with society's dominant rationales, power relations and social norms (see Chap. 2), unless they are embedded in broader health promotion strategies, that is, a strategy that addresses the economic, spatial and political structures of life worlds and settings (e.g. the neighbourhood, workplace or school).

In contrast to such comprehensive approaches, the mission and commitment of International Life Science Institute (ILSI), as a globally active 'astroturf non-profit' organisation, is paradigmatic. ILSI cooperates with governments in order to co-produce scientific evidence. The organisation's primary goal is to prevent industry being subjected to restrictive regulations (see Chap. 5) and—meanwhile—it has also been developing 'behavioural health governance' in order to achieve its aims. While the challenge posed by NCDs is growing steadily and exponentially and requires an immediate response, this kind of 'public-private partnerships of evidence-based policymaking' are likely to pull the global framework for health promotion and disease prevention in the future in a particular direction. As a consequence, area-based and cross-sectoral approaches that struggle to achieve structural changes (i.e. taming the influence of the food industry) may become further side-lined due to the 'raw politics' (Raphael 2014) that make it difficult to pursue a truly comprehensive public health strategy. As such, the complexity dilemma of public health is far from resolved, even if 'simplified experimental logics and simple solutions' (Chap. 4) create the contrary impression. Behavioural insights sometimes make it appear as if solutions in public health can be found easily. However, a closer inspection reveals that behavioural insights, if applied in a comprehensive manner, also have the potential to accommodate complexity. Notwithstanding, as set out by Pykett in this book (Chap. 4), political, economic and cultural contexts cannot be circumvented by behavioural interventions but provide a breeding ground in which country-specific amalgams of health policies (which consist of instrument mixes) can emerge and develop. To arrive at a more nuanced picture, it is necessary to explore in greater empirical depth the contextual differences concerning the effects of behavioural health policies. In this regard, it is not only interesting whether 'Europeans support health nudges' (Reisch and Sunstein 2016) but also how behavioural instruments interconnect with the legacies of previous policy and institutional heritage in the field of health promotion. It does not require too much analytical acumen to predict that the question of whether behavioural interventions are applied within liberal welfare states (like the UK and the US) or within classic European welfare states, will play a significant role. For instance, the heated debate on choice architectures in school cafeterias could be viewed in a different light if 'smart lunchrooms' (Wansink 2016) are embedded in a 'thick' (i.e. more generous) welfare state, such as that of Finland, where families have access to state-funded health counselling and where school meals are free of charge and certified as healthy (Ewert 2017a). Similarly, bicycle-friendly European cities such as Amsterdam and Copenhagen are viewed less through the health promotion lens and, primarily, as role models for smart city planning. In short, it makes a significant difference whether health nudges are viewed as a panacea within political and economic structures that are otherwise offer relatively little in the way of support for public health (and in which the likelihood of people suffering from NCDs is relatively high), or whether the use of nudges is viewed as one of a range of intelligent policy instruments within a multi-dimensional health promotion strategy.

Rather than downplaying the potential of behavioural tools in health promotion, this finding brings us again to the question of where and when policies should be informed by behavioural insights. Opinions on this awkward question vary widely in the relatively new academic discourse on 'nudging in public policy' (Van Deun et al. 2018). Unsurprisingly, this is also mirrored by the arguments concerning the future role of behavioural techniques gathered within this book. Ewert (Chap. 2) and Loer (Chap. 3) are slightly optimistic that behavioural insights could be carefully integrated into existing health policies and, hence, may address public health issues more comprehensively. Instead Pykett (Chap. 4) remains sceptical that nudging, at least in its sudden use, bear the potential to face challenges such as health inequality that is caused by the 'dynamic relation between place and people's health'. Moreover, Loer and Strassheim (Chap. 5) remind us that, if not negotiated in the public realm and politically legitimised, strategies of behavioural governance may not fit common interest. Hitherto, as demonstrated by the cases studies in this book, behavioural policies have been mainly restricted to the implementation of health promotion measures and thus to end-users' choice-making behaviour, which has been meticulously explored under laboratory conditions in advance. However, 'introducing a more realistic model of human behaviour to policy' (BIT 2018), one of the main objectives of UK's Behavioural Insight Team (BIT) could also be applied in a more reflexive manner to the process of policymaking itself, that is, to any stage and actor within it. What may sound like a utopian or even rather naïve idea at first glance, could, if operationalised effectively, be a useful approach to nudging 'departments in applying cross-government agendas' (OECD 2017, 50), as suggested by health-in-all-policies approaches (Leppo et al. 2013). Moreover, behavioural insights may facilitate multi-professional cooperation and teamwork in health-promoting settings that often face an implementation deficit in practice due to unforeseen (i.e. non-compliant) behaviour by policy stakeholders. This is this area where the potential of behavioural policy interventions remains untapped.

Implications of Behavioural Health Policies for Citizens

The second point to discuss in this conclusion concerns the implications for citizens' rights and responsibilities within a behaviourally informed policy environment in public health. Under the paradigm of behavioural health policies, the concept of 'health citizenship' (Huisman and Oosterhuis 2014), which has emerged in (mainly Western) welfare states, has to be reassessed. Traditionally, health citizenship has been marked by the trinity of confidence in the state, institutions and professions, but also by free choice in lifestyles and healthcare provision, as well as voice in relation to healthcare professionals and within the process of health policy-making (e.g. in corporatist health regimes). In health promotion, enjoying health citizenship has traditionally meant, on the one hand, the steady proliferation of state protection against the most obvious health risks with regard to living and working conditions. On the other hand, citizens have been perceived, as claimed in the Ottawa Charter, as social agents who seek 'ownership and control of their own endeavours and destinies' (WHO 1986) in their various life worlds. Thus, achieving optimal physical and mental health requires environmental cues that empower people to live healthier lives (rather than coercing them to do so) as well as opportunities for voice and participation. In this sense, maintaining individual health means much more than merely pursuing a health-promoting lifestyle, that is, being happy, eating well and being physically active. Rather, it necessitates a positive attitude towards life that fosters learning and includes the ability to socialise with others and engage beyond one's own immediate interests. When understood this way, health citizenship, in relation to health promotion, is of course a highly ambitious goal, which reality is probably destined to fall short of.

The rise of behavioural policymaking that primarily addresses errant humans, rather than responsible citizens, has implications for health citizenship as a concept in health promotion. There are a number of pressing questions in this regard. Can institutional trust be maintained if citizens are (stealthily) nudged by the 'behaviour change state' (Leggett 2014, 4)? What is the value of individual choice if policymakers openly and unambiguously promote their view of what a socially desirable healthy lifestyle looks like? And how can we deal with citizens' voice and agency if choice architects unilaterally answer crucial questions such as 'Who decides? Which nudges are applied? Regarding which forms of behaviour? Based on which minimum level of evidence?' (Brown 2012, 313). It seems beyond question that behavioural policies in health promotion will challenge the traditional hallmarks of health citizenship. With regard to institutional trust, much depends on the nature of the (welfare) state that applies behavioural insights in health promotion. Nudge advocates remind governments to 'nudge for good' (Thaler 2015), while citizens consider nudging to be a legitimate approach in cases where they feel that 'it fits with the interests and value of most people' (Reisch and Sunstein 2016, 322). However, such a pledge of confidence may soon become exhausted if governments' appetite for behavioural policymaking coincides with a period of extended fiscal austerity and welfare retrenchment. Nudged citizens may wonder whether behavioural interventions are actually the most effective policy tools available, or simply the cheapest. They may also wonder if it is not the state's noble task to protect its citizens in the face of behavioural assaults by an 'army' of unprincipled nudgers from the commercial sector. In addition, public trust in state-driven behaviourally informed health policies may be significantly undermined if citizens become aware that the scientific evidence of behavioural interventions has been co-created by industry-friendly non-profits such as ILSI (see Chap. 5). Furthermore, ongoing digitalisation is creating other sensitive issues in relation to institutional trust. Health-related data concerning, for example, people's driving style or exercise routines, may, if not carefully protected, come to be used systematically by insurance companies and state agencies to nudge specific target groups with 'behavioural abnormalities'. In this regard, the dystopian plan of the Chinese government to introduce a digital 'citizen rating' that is based on citizens' past behaviour gives us a hint what sort of behavioural governance, using digitally available data, may become possible in near future (Botsman 2017).

If confidence in the state is further undermined through behavioural health policies, the implications for the citizen's right to choice in relation to their own lifestyle are more nuanced. In general, citizens' choice of lifestyle is not restricted by modified choice architectures; one could even argue that the application of behavioural tools that support citizens' well-being may increase their freedom to choose lifestyles that they may well have reason to value. Since there are good reasons that health represents an intrinsic value for most people, it is perfectly reasonable to argue that health nudges and other behavioural instruments do not restrict choice, but 'leave freedom of choice' (Schmidt 2017, 408). However, the inherent problem of behaviourally informed health promotion strategies is the extent to which certain public values and social norms become entrenched. Health nudges that prompt us to, for example, eat vegetables instead of potato fries, to stay physically active and to avoid being sedentary, collide on a more general level with pluralistic societies in which citizens' attitudes towards health 'may interfere with interests representing other aspects of the good life' (White 2016, 76). Viewed this way, the behavioural change state may not become a rigid nanny state (Le Grand and New 2015) but a (more or less) moralising and patronising agency that bestows a 'subtle stigma' (Eyal 2014, 54) on those who choose unhealthier lifestyles.

Finally, the question arises of how citizens' voice and participation may change through behavioural health policies. It would seem that health nudges and the like address active rather than passive citizens; in addition, the success of those interventions depends on the degree to which citizens actually utilise the behavioural cues sent out by health policymakers. It is theoretically conceivable that behavioural policies may be the result of a deliberative bottom-up process, in which active citizens take joint decisions on health promotion strategies, that is, its means and goals (see the concept of a 'behaviourally informed health citizenship' below). Seen from this angle, behaviourally informed health governance would not contradict the key principle of the Ottawa Charter for Health Promotion, according to which citizens ought to be 'able to take decisions and have control over [their] life circumstances' (WHO 1986). For example, under the settings approach, behavioural insights could be used to achieve health promotion goals that have been defined through deliberation in advance—as suggested in theoretical discussions of combining 'nudge' and 'think' strategies (John et al. 2009). Likewise, Schmidt (2017, 411) has convincingly argued 'that it is feasible to place nudge policies under suitable democratic control', particularly 'in local institutions (such as schools)'. However, empirical evidence on the successful implementation of 'democratically controlled' behavioural policies in health promotion remains almost absent (see Feitsma 2018 for an exception). Instead, health nudges that have been developed top-down continue to dominate and may come to dominate still further, given corporate efforts to influence behavioural policymaking (see the example of ILSI). As a consequence, we must take seriously the risk that the active engagement of citizens may be reduced to compliance with the intentions of a rather elitist form of behavioural health governance. If thought through to its logical end-point, such a policy approach could lead to an impoverished meaning of health citizenship, because it does not foster civic virtues such as voice and collective action within the practice of health promotion (Ewert 2017b).

Towards a Behaviourally Informed Health Citizenship

Behavioural policies are accompanied by great hopes of innovative solutions for wicked problems such as NCDs. At the same time, there is a great deal of criticism and distrust concerning the systematic use of behavioural insights in policymaking, mainly voiced by social scientists with concerns about 'a less deliberately oriented and rational self (...) which is likely to be reinforced by related forms of disempowering behavioural government' (Whitehead et al. 2018, 93). This holds especially true in the field of health promotion, which, by tradition, has been closely linked to citizenship's core elements such as empowerment, community-building and collective action. However, rather than joining in with the chorus that dismisses behavioural health policies as an insidious new form of governmentality (Jones et al. 2013), we will close this book by making the argument for a reconciliation between citizenship and behavioural governance as suggested by a 'behaviourally-informed health citizenship' (see also Ewert 2018). Given the limited space that we have here, we can only provide the bare bones of such a concept. Nevertheless, sketching out three essential features that would characterise a behaviourally informed health citizenship will allow us to move beyond the supposed dichotomy between citizen rights in the field of health and health promotion and recent approaches to behavioural health governance.

First, a behaviourally informed health citizenship concept ought to provide clarity on the exact role of citizens' behaviour in health promotion policies. Of necessity, a general consensus must be established that 'behaviour' is the result of, and is constrained by 'structures' (Spotswood and Marsh 2016, 286); consequently, behavioural change requires, above all, structural interventions rather than simply focusing on 'the 'doers' of behaviour' (ibid.). Health nudges that regulate the built environment to increase physical activity fit into this category without reducing citizens to subjects with behavioural problems.

Second, building on the first feature of a behaviourally informed health citizenship, citizens ought to have the right to protection against the unchallenged 'power of private companies to nudge' (Schmidt 2017, 413). On the one hand, this will require new forms of regulation in as-yet unregulated areas. A timely example of the latter are social media channels where vulnerable groups such as children and teenagers are exposed to subtle but perfectly targeted advertising for unhealthy products and lifestyles. On the other hand, the adoption of a standardised traffic light system for food labelling and an intelligent calorie-labelling system would help to put health-conscious citizens in a much stronger position in the 'battleground' of behavioural change. If at all possible in advanced capitalist societies, such examples of 'public nudges' (ibid.) would actually help citizens 'to become risk savvy' (Gigerenzer 2015, 361).

Third, if applied consistently as part of a comprehensive approach to health promotion, behavioural instruments need to be 'transparent and democratically controlled' (Schmidt 2017, 404). Citizens ought to be able to recognise when they are being nudged within the public realm (Bovens 2009) and, thus, be given the right to deliberate and decide over the context, form and goal of nudges. Within people's life worlds and the setting of a democratic society, it is feasible to fulfil both criteria (Schmidt 2017). By way of example, local policy boards could confirm nudges that promote walkability within neighbourhoods; likewise, students could co-design the choice architecture in their school cafeteria.

At has been demonstrated throughout this book, the debate on and the use of behavioural insights has breathed new life into the art of policymaking in health promotion. Viewed pragmatically, as a complement to conventional policy instruments (John 2013) and simply adding a behavioural spin (Loer forthcoming), behavioural interventions are unquestionably an enrichment—another arrow in the policymaker's quiver. Nevertheless, whether behaviourally informed policies will turn out to be successful in the fight against public health challenges such as NCDs today depends more than ever on collective actions to improve the social determinants of health. Hence, for the field of health promotion, the really intriguing question for the near future will be whether behaviourally informed health policies have the potential to bridge the 'chasm between two central views' (Baum and Fisher 2014, 214) on how to promote health. In short, can behavioural policies reduce health inequalities by promoting health at the individual level as well as at the structural level? Ideally, and hopefully, the future use of behavioural insights will contribute to, rather than exacerbate, this unfinished business in health promotion and disease prevention.

References

Baum, F., & Fisher, M. (2014). Why behavioural health promotion endures despite its failure to reduce health inequities. *Sociology of Health & Illness, 36*(2), 213–225.

Behavioural Insight Team (BIT). (2018). *Who we are*. Retrieved February 26, 2018, from http://www.behaviouralinsights.co.uk/about-us/

Botsman, R. (2017). *Who can you trust?: How technology brought us together and why it might drive us apart*. New York: Public Affairs.

Bovens, L. (2009). The ethics of nudge. In T. Grüne-Yanoff & S. O. Hansson (Eds.), *Preference change: Approaches from philosophy, economics and psychology* (pp. 207–220). Dordrecht: Springer.

Brown, P. (2012). A nudge in the right direction? Towards a sociological engagement with libertarian paternalism. *Social Policy and Society, 11*, 305–317.
Butland, B., Jebb, S., Kopelman, P., McPherson, K., Thomas, S., Mardell, J., & Parry, V. (2007). Foresight. In *Tackling obesities: Future choices – Project report.* London: Government Office for Science.
Clavier, C., & de Leeuw, E. (2013). *Health promotion and the policy process.* Oxford: Oxford University Press.
Crawshaw, P. (2013). Public health policy and the behavioural turn: The case of social marketing. *Critical Social Policy, 33*(4), 616–637.
de Leeuw, E., & Peters, D. (2014). Nine questions to guide development and implementation of health in all policies. *Health Promotion International, 30*(4). https://doi.org/10.1093/heapro/dau034.
Dooris, M. (2009). Holistic and sustainable health improvement: The contribution of the settings-based approach to health promotion. *Perspectives in Public Health, 129*(1), 29–36.
Ewert, B. (2017a). *A Gallic Village that bucked the trend of childhood obesity: Report on a study trip to Seinäjoki (Finland).* Retrieved March 9, 2018, from https://hse.hypotheses.org/554
Ewert, B. (2017b). Promoting health in schools: Theoretical reflections on the settings approach versus nudge tactics. *Social Theory & Health, 15*(4), 430–447.
Ewert, B. (2018). From entitled citizens to nudged consumers? Re-examining the hallmarks of health citizenship in the light of the behavioural turn. *Public Policy and Administration, 0*(0), 1–21. https://doi.org/10.1177/0952076718774612.
Eyal, N. (2014). Nudging by shaming, shaming by nudging. *International Journal of Health Policy Management, 3*(2), 53–56.
Feitsma, J. N. P. (2018). The behavioural state: Critical observations on technocracy and psychocracy. *Policy Sciences, 51*(3), 387–410.
Gigerenzer, G. (2015). On the supposed evidence for libertarian paternalism. *Review of Philosophy and Psychology, 6*(3), 361–383.
Huisman, F., & Oosterhuis, F. (2014). *Health and citizenship: Political cultures of health in modern Europe.* London: Pickering & Chatto.
John, P. (2013). All tools are informational now: How information and persuasion define the tools of government. *Policy & Politics, 41*(4), 605–620.
John, P., Smith, G., & Stroker, G. (2009). Nudge nudge, think think: Two strategies of changing civic behaviour. *The Political Quarterly, 80*(3), 361–370.
Jones, R., Pykett, J., & Whitehead, M. (2013). Psychological governance and behaviour change. *Policy & Politics, 41*(2), 159–182.
Le Grand, J., & New, B. (2015). *Government paternalism nanny state or helpful friend?* Princeton: Princeton University Press.
Leggett, W. (2014). The politics of behaviour change: Nudge, neoliberalism and the state. *Policy & Politics, 42*(1), 3–19.
Leppo, K., Ollila, E., Peña, S., Wismar, M., & Cook, S. (2013). Health in all policies. In *Seizing opportunities, implementing policies.* Helsinki: Ministry of Social Affairs and Health, Finland.

Loer, K. (forthcoming). The enzymatic effect of behavioural sciences – What about policy-maker's expectations? In S. Beck & H. Strassheim (Eds.), *Handbook on behavioural change and public policy*. Cheltenham: Edward Elgar.

Marmot, M. (2005). Social determinants of health inequalities. *Lancet, 365*(9464), 1099–1104.

OECD. (2017). *Behavioural insights and public policy: Lessons from around the world*. Paris: OECD Publishing.

Raphael, D. (2014). Beyond policy analysis: The raw politics behind opposition to healthy public policy. *Health Promotion International, 30*(2), 380–396.

Reisch, L. A., & Sunstein, C. R. (2016). Do European like nudges? *Judgment and Decision making, 11*(4), 310–325.

Schmidt, A. T. (2017). The power to nudge. *American Political Science Review, 111*(2), 404–417.

Spotswood, F., & Marsh, A. (2016). Conclusion: What is the future of 'behaviour change'? In F. Spotswood (Ed.), *Beyond behaviour change. Key issues, interdisciplinary approaches and future directions* (pp. 283–298). Bristol: Policy Press.

Thaler, R. H. (2015, October 31). The power of nudges, for good and bad. *The New York Times* (Economic View).

Van Deun, H., van Acker, W., Fobé, E., & Brans, M. (2018, March 26–28). *Nudging in public policy and public management: A scoping review of the literature*. Presented at the Political Studies Association 68th Annual International Conference, Cardiff University. Retrieved June 4, 2018, from https://www.psa.ac.uk/sites/default/files/conference/papers/2018/VanDeun_vanAcker_Fobé_Brans_Nudging_Scoping%20Review.pdf

Wansink, B. (2016). Slim by design: Moving from can't to can. In C. A. Roberto & I. Kawachi (Eds.), *Behavioral economics and public health* (pp. 237–264). Oxford: Oxford University Press.

White, M. D. (2016). Bad medicine: Does the unique nature of healthcare decisions justify nudges? In G. I. Cohen, H. F. Lynch, & C. T. Robertson (Eds.), *Nudging health: Health law and behavioral economics* (pp. 72–82). Baltimore: John Hopkins University Press.

Whitehead, M., Jones, R., Lilley, R., Pykett, J., & Howell, R. (2018). *Neuroliberalism. Behavioural government in the twenty-first century*. London/New York: Routledge.

WHO. (1986). *Ottawa Charter for health promotion*. Retrieved December 29, 2017, from http://www.euro.who.int/__data/assets/pdf_file/0004/129532/Ottawa_Charter.pdf?ua=1

Index[1]

[1]Note: Page numbers followed by 'n' refer to notes.

B. Ewert, K. Loer (eds.), *Behavioural Policies for Health Promotion and Disease Prevention*, Palgrave Studies in Public Health Policy Research, https://doi.org/10.1007/978-3-319-98316-5

The manufacturer's authorised representative in the EU is Springer Nature Customer Service Centre GmbH, Europaplatz 3, 69115 Heidelberg, Germany. If you have any concerns regarding our products, please contact ProductSafety@springernature.com

Printed and bound by CPI Group (UK) Ltd, Croydon, CR0 4YY
22/09/2026
02221067-0013